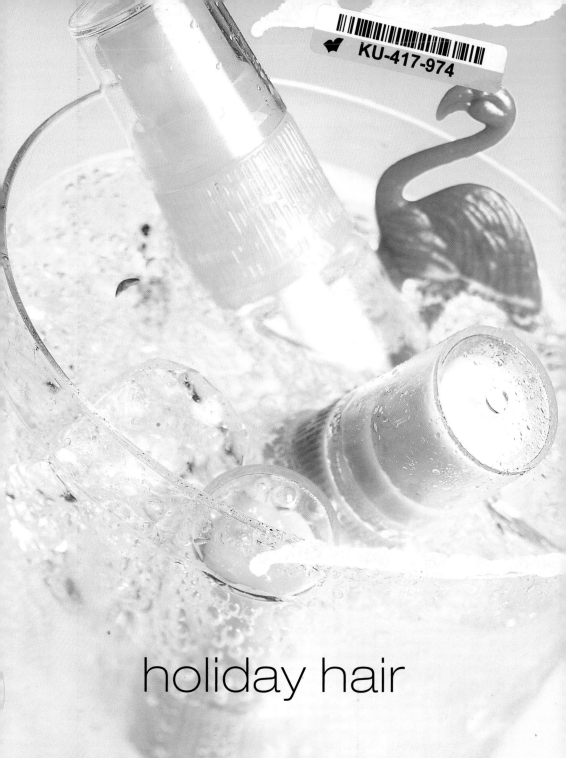

holiday hair

THIS IS A CARLTON BOOK

Design, text and photography copyright © 2001 Carlton Books Limited
Original idea and concept copyright © 2001 Charles Worthington Limited

This edition published by Carlton Books Limited 2001
20 Mortimer Street
London W1T 3JW

A CIP catalogue record for this book is available from the British Library

ISBN paperback 1 84222 199 X
ISBN hardback 1 84222 257 0

The author, licensor and publisher have made every effort to ensure that all information is correct and up to date at the time of publication. Neither the author, licensor or publisher can accept responsibility for any accident, injury or damage that results from using the ideas, information or advice offered.

The application and quality of hair products and treatments, herbal preparations and essential oils is beyond the control of the above parties, who cannot be held responsible for any problems resulting from their use. Always follow the manufacturer's instructions and, if in doubt, seek further advice.

Do not use herbal preparations or essential oils without prior consultation with a qualified practitioner or medical doctor if you are pregnant, taking any form of medication, or if you suffer from oversensitive skin. Half-doses of essential oils should always be used for children and the elderly.

No resemblance is intended to any person, living or dead, in the fiction element of this book. The events and the characters who take part in them have no relation to actual events or living people.

Writer: Emma Craven, Beauty Editor, *Red*
Photographer (model): Hugh Arnold
Photographer (still life): Patrice de Villiers
Illustrator: Jason Brooks
Stylist: Rachel Davis
Make-up: Chase Aston
Editorial Manager: Venetia Penfold
Art Director: Penny Stock
Senior Art Editor: Barbara Zuñiga
Commissioning Editor: Zia Mattocks
Production Controller: Janette Davis

Printed and bound in Italy

holiday hair

Charles Worthington

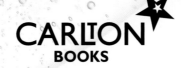

contents

foreword

Holiday's are a great time to experiment with new styling ideas and hair products – after all, you're in a different place, with people you'll probably never see again in your life, so go for it! Try those dreadlocks or that glamorous big, big hairstyle that you've always longed for! But be warned: holidays can also be very damaging to the hair if you don't look after it properly and take all the necessary precautions. A change of climate – whether hot and dry, humid or cold – can cause all manner of hair disasters, from fading colour to split ends. This book covers your every need for healthy, gorgeous holiday hair. It will help you prep your hair before you go away, so that whatever your destination, your hair will be easy to manage and looking its best. In addition, there are lots of fantastic styling ideas for great holiday looks, whether you're heading for the ski slopes, the beach, a spa retreat or a city. There's also advice on how to get your hair back in peak conditon when you get home. So, whatever your choice of holiday reading, don't forget to pack this book in your suitcase!

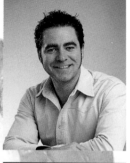

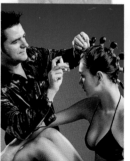

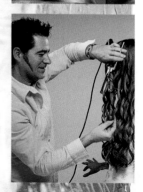

Charles Worthington

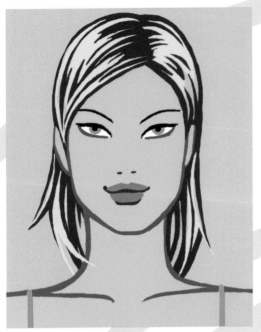

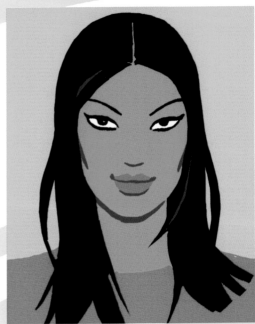

polly

Polly is a City career babe – traditional, yes, but she's got a twist. Her double first in maths means she can tot up her buying splurges as fast as the computers at Visa. She always looks immaculate and only her closest friends know that her sleek blonde hair is the result of painstaking styling to iron out its natural wave. A sexy new man on the scene – American cyber-suitor Simon – has given Polly a new lease of life and looks. He's literally swept her off her feet and the time has come to wave goodbye to unappreciative and rather dull Harry.

jaz

Jaz (short for Jasmine) is your regular club bunnie. She loves all things hip, cool and girlie. Her earliest memory is of dressing up in the contents of her mother's overstuffed wardrobe – and clothes are still her greatest passion. She can't remember the last time she took off her make-up before going to bed but, with her long, thick, glossy black hair, she always looks stunning nevertheless. Jaz has finally landed her dream job as fashion assistant at *Gloss* magazine, which has further fuelled her passion for fashion and new hairstyles.

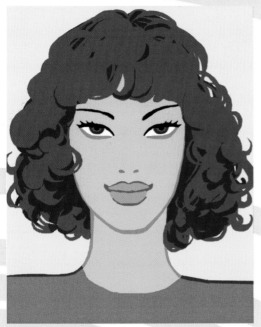

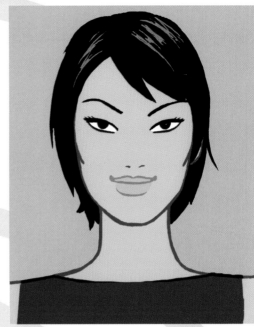

kate

Kate looks like a pre-Raphaelite painting: unruly curly titian hair, milky complexion and rosy cheeks. She works as a personal assistant to the marketing director of Crunch Biscuits – not a good career choice when you have a sweet tooth and are prone to overindulgence. A hopeless romantic with an insatiable – and unrequited – crush on her boss, Kate has decided that it's time to make some serious changes in her life. It's not just her looks and love life that are in need of a revamp, her career needs something of a kick-start, too.

laura

Laura is a tomboy: lean and androgynous with a short crop. Her uniform is urban cool – more combats and trainers than pencil skirts and kitten heels. She's a struggling TV researcher who wants to make gritty documentaries and dreams of winning a BAFTA. Her redefined image – still tomboy but with a feminine twist – has surprised both herself and the other girls. It's not entirely coincidental, though; she's been trying to attract the attention of a certain assistant TV producer, John, for simply ages – and it looks like it might not have gone unnoticed.

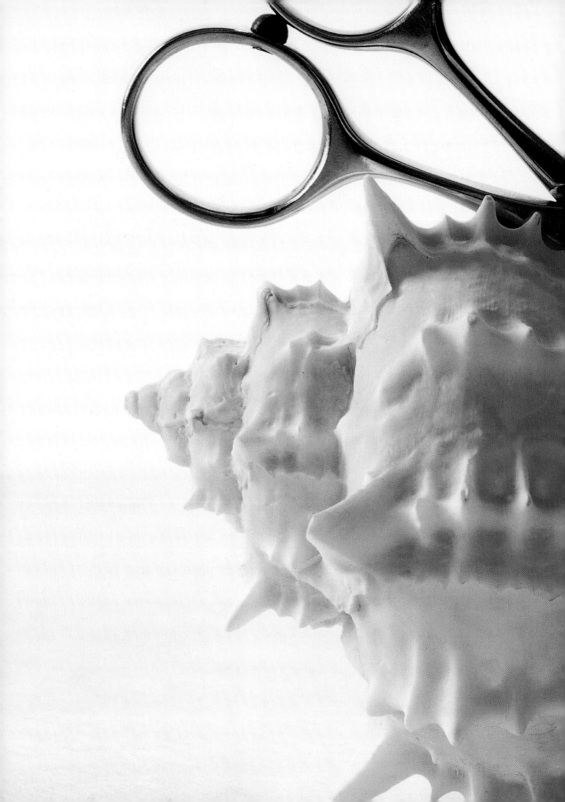

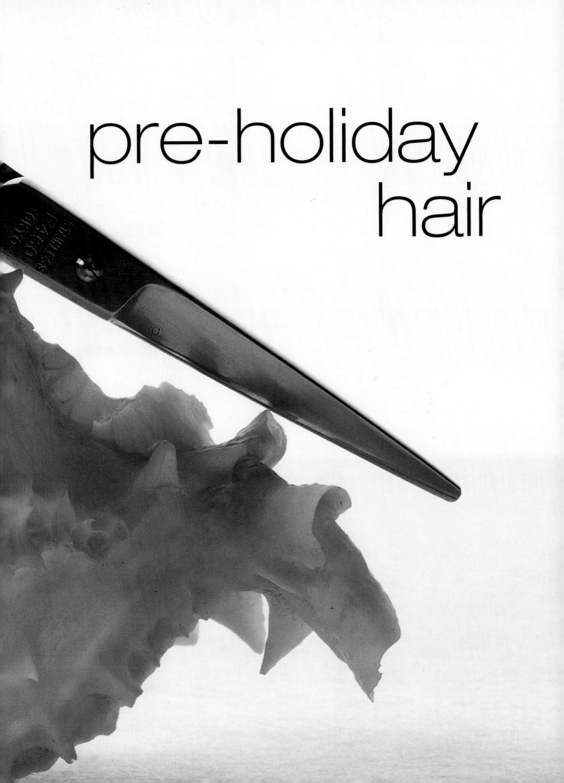

pre-holiday
hair

morning after the big date night

'So how long have you been seeing him?' asked Chrissie, the girls' house guest from New York (who now seemed to be a permanent fixture, having originally planned to stay for a month). She'd been dying to know all the details since spotting 'perfect' Polly with a gorgeous man in Cirque the night before. The girls were draped across the sofa in their sitting room, feeling worse for wear after their big night out.

'Since New York,' Polly admitted. She'd been bursting to tell the girls about her cyber-suitor, Simon, since their affair had started. And now the secret was out. 'Are you planning to tell Harry?' demanded Chrissie. How ridiculous of Chrissie to take the moral viewpoint, thought Polly. If she'd met someone as perfect as Simon she wouldn't be letting him go in a hurry. 'I'm going to tell him at dinner,' answered Polly. 'Though I have to say, Chrissie, I thought you'd support me on this. Simon's everything I've been looking for in a boyfriend, everything Harry isn't. I'm sure he's the one.' 'How about finishing one relationship before you start another?' Chrissie snapped.

Chrissie was smarting with jealousy. Despite her careful preening and fabulous outfit, Steve had barely noticed her. It was obvious that his attention was fixed on Laura. To make matters worse, Steve's friend John, who was supposed to be Chrissie's blind date, turned out to be Laura's work colleague. It was clear from John's enthusiasm and Laura's flirting that they were keen on each other. Chrissie could hardly believe it – two gorgeous men competing over Laura! Chrissie was used to being the centre of attention and yet last night no one had seemed interested in talking to her. Now she could tell that Polly was bursting to talk about Simon and how they had got together, but Chrissie's hurt ego had got the better of her. The details of Polly's affair would have to wait; the two girls fell into a tense silence.

Upstairs, Laura was just waking up. She lay in bed for a while thinking over every detail of last night. She'd nearly fallen off her kitten heels when she'd discovered that Steve's single friend was John, the sexy assistant TV producer at work. The rest of the evening had been fantastic. Her flirty hairstyle and feminine clothes had done the trick – not only had Steve been drooling over her all evening, but John had made it clear that he was interested in more than work chat. In fact, he'd asked for her number before she left the club and she'd watched him write it on a card and carefully tuck it into his wallet. Laura was delighted with herself. She'd played her part perfectly all night: flirty and interesting but just that little bit unavailable at the same time. She smiled to herself. 'He'll call me,' she thought, 'he won't be able to resist.'

In her executive hotel room, Kate was suffering with a hangover and crushed confidence. She'd felt so sure of herself when she was getting dressed for the Crunch Ball the night before. Entering the ballroom, she'd caught the eye of her boss, Matthew, and his double take had given her a rush. 'You look really … great,' he'd managed to say. But just as she'd begun her carefully planned, bright and engaging conversation, Rachel, a leggy brunette from the sales division, had slipped her arm through Matthew's and pulled him towards her. Cutting into Kate's conversation mid-sentence, Rachel had looked her up and down patronizingly and said, 'You don't mind do you Kate? Matthew and I have got some important figures to discuss.' Without a backward glance, Matthew had walked off with Rachel giggling on his arm. The rest of the evening had been a complete nightmare. Kate had decided to drown her sorrows with complimentary champagne, and she'd looked hot and dishevelled by the time she reached her room later that night.

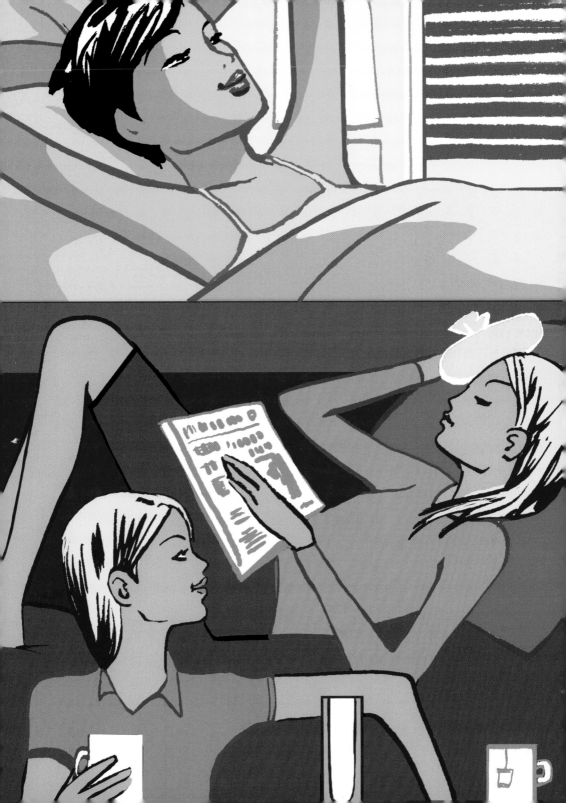

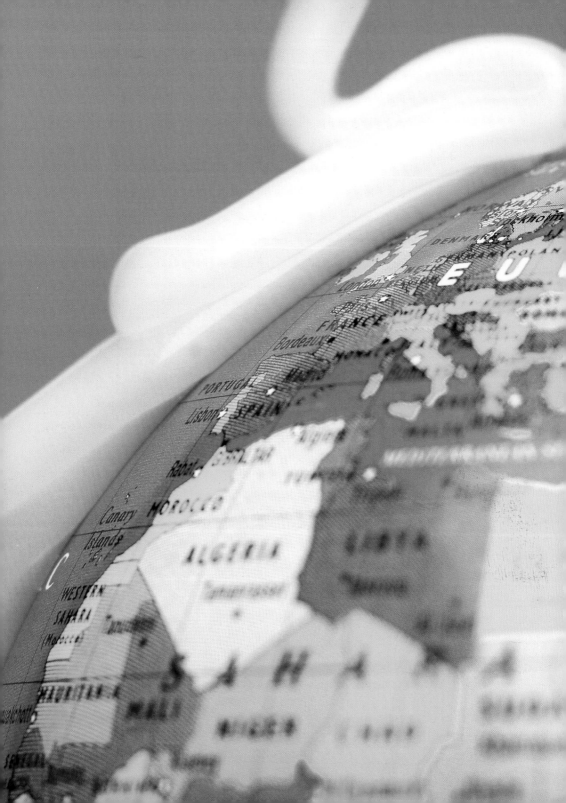

going away

Each year we look forward to our holidays and dream of sun-drenched days, relaxation and the chance to indulge ourselves, pushing our holiday budgets to the limit. We buy new clothes, cosmetics and perfume to look our best while we are away and often leave our haircare to the last minute. Foreign travel – whether it's to a hot destination for some sun, sandy beaches and clear blue sea or to the mountains to enjoy fresh air and crisp snow – will always be good for recharging your batteries, but rarely good for your hair. On holiday you are going to be miles away from your usual hair salon and the creature comforts of your own bathroom. However laid-back you might want to be on holiday, it's likely that there will be moments when you want your hair to look its best. And whatever the climate of your destination, you will probably be outside your usual environment and, as a result, your hair will be under attack from weather that it's not used to.

Your hair, unlike your skin, has no natural defence system. The ultraviolet (UV) rays of the sun, even on a relatively cloudy day, beat down on your head and dry out your hair. UV rays create free radicals, which attack the hair within the hair shaft as well as on its surface. The pigments within the hair (which give hair its colour) are damaged by the sun, and daily exposure breaks down the hair's strength, causing a loss in colour intensity, shine and vitality. So, when you are away, you should try to think of your haircare routine in the same way as you do your skincare routine. When you go on holiday, you pack a cleanser, moisturizer and sun-protection and after-sun lotions for your face; your hair needs similar treatment. Shampoo, conditioner, sunscreen for hair and a styling product should all make it into your wash-bag. You should condition colour-treated hair after every wash – at home or on holiday. Uncoloured hair should be conditioned when you are away to prevent damage from the new environment. Remember, you cannot over-condition your hair. Just choose a conditioner to suit your hair type, be it fine and flyaway or thick and curly.

cold climate

Cold weather makes hair very brittle and can cause dryness. The effect on the hair is just as if you were to climb into a refrigerator and cool your hair down extremely quickly – it leaves it weakened and vulnerable to damage. Low temperatures can also cause static or flyaway hair and this is a particular problem for fine hair types, especially those with poker-straight hair. Many people tend to rough-dry their hair, leaving it slightly damp, and simply tie it back before going outside – a definite no-no for hair in the cold. Keep your hair well conditioned if you are spending time in low temperatures and, whenever possible, wear a hat to keep your hair from exposure to the cold.

fine hair

Use a gentle, everyday shampoo and a light, leave-in conditioner to keep the ends of your hair protected. In extremely low temperatures, always use a heat-protection spray before styling, and work some serum sparingly through the ends of the hair after blow-drying to seal the hair shaft and lock the moisture in. If you find your hair becomes static, spray a little hairspray onto your brush and smooth down the flyaway hair.

curly hair

A good conditioning treatment after shampooing your hair helps to keep your tresses shiny and well conditioned. Again, a heat-protection spray is a must, plus serum after blow-drying to keep the hair hydrated.

frizzy hair

This tends to be much drier than other hair types. Use a leave-in conditioner after shampooing and take a deep-moisturizing mask with you on holiday to give the hair an intensive treatment at least twice a week. A heat-protection spray and hair serum will keep the moisture locked into your tresses and keep the elements out.

humid climate

Whatever your hair type, your hair swells and expands when it's wet and behaves in the same way in a humid climate, where the air is full of moisture. Humidity will make hair fluffy and, if it's prone to curling, it will cause frizziness. All hair types will benefit from a pre-holiday conditioning treatment in the salon to nourish the hair shafts and seal the cuticles. Preventing excess moisture from entering the hair shaft in a humid climate is key.

fine hair

This tends to get weighed down by the moisture in the air and looks flat and limp. Just as with other hair types, you need to block out the humidity if you can. A pre-holiday salon treatment will help to reduce split ends and close the cuticles that allow water to enter the hair shaft. Use a light leave-in conditioner on your hair while you are away (apply it from mid-way down the length of your hair to the ends) and seal the ends of the hair after blow-drying with a serum. Be careful not to use too much serum on fine hair – a blob the size of your thumbnail is more than enough. Hairsprays are a great SOS option for a bad-hair day in humidity – they instantly hold down the cuticle of the hair and prevent moisture from entering the hair shaft.

curly and frizzy hair

Sealing the outside of your hair – the cuticle – is the only way you will minimize the candyfloss look while you are away. A pre-holiday deep-conditioning treatment is a must. Make sure you pack a creamy leave-in conditioner for your trip and use it religiously every morning. Using an anti-frizz serum will help bring unruly curls to heel. It coats the hair shaft with silicone, not only sealing the cuticle but also weighing the hair down a little. If your hair is really frizzy, try working some serum through it while it is still wet before blow-drying. This should add some weight to the curls and seal the cuticles so that your hair does not absorb water, swell and frizz again as it dries. If you decide to go with the flow and make the most of your curls while you're away, mix gel and serum together in the palm of your hand and apply it throughout the hair to give the curls extra definition and shape.

hot, dry heat

The sun can strip the hair of its natural oils and a dry heat will only intensify the problem. Just two weeks in the sun without protecting your hair can weaken hair cuticles, with peeling, breaking and split ends becoming a problem. The sun's UV rays attack the melanin pigment that gives hair its colour, as well as the keratin, the protein fibres, within the hair shaft that provide strength and elasticity. A weakened cuticle leaves hair vulnerable to dehydration and the colour bleaches and fades. Sun exposure also encourages free radical activity in the hair shaft. The cells of the hair are damaged, as the free radicals cause premature ageing. Deep-conditioning treatments are vital before travelling to a hot climate, especially for chemically treated hair. However, the only way to protect your hair 100 per cent from sun damage is to keep it out of the sun – a hat is the best option.

fine hair

Pack a gentle daily shampoo and a light leave-in conditioner with UV protection. A sun-protection spray that contains a UV filter will help screen the hair from the sun and sea water if you are sunbathing on a beach. Reapply the spray through the hair after each dip in the sea.

curly hair

Pack a gentle moisturizing shampoo to cleanse your hair daily, plus a creamy leave-in conditioner to help guard against excess dryness. If you are sunbathing, apply a sun-protection spray or oil that contains a UV filter to reduce sun damage to the hair, and reapply it regularly, just as you would suntan lotion to your face and body. Take a nourishing hair mask with you to deep-condition your hair.

frizzy hair

Your hair tends to be dry anyway and needs extra care in dry heat. As before, use a sun-protection spray or oil on your hair during the day and make sure you apply a rich leave-in conditioner with UV protection to your hair each morning before going out in the sun. Apply a hair mask to your hair at least every other day during your holiday – you can leave it on overnight for an intensive treatment if your hair becomes very dry in the heat.

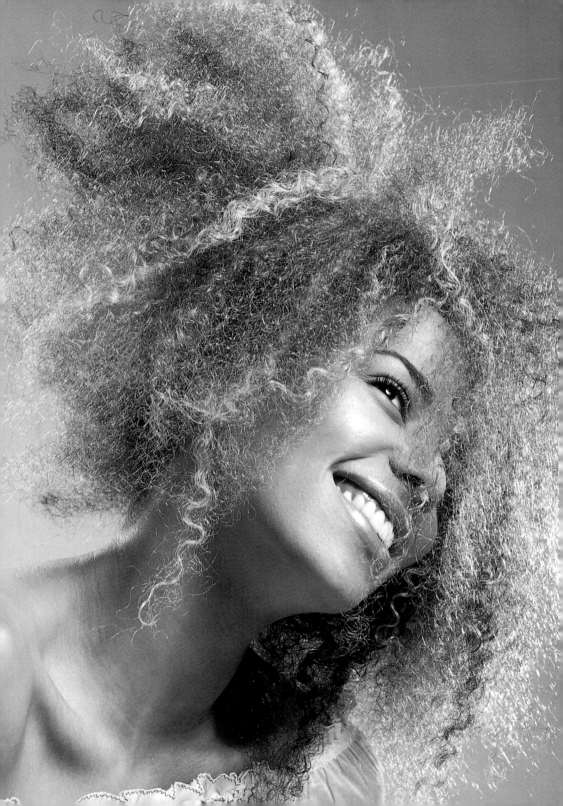

holiday hair enemies

All weather and climate changes bring environmental aggressors that are damaging to your hair. The perfect holiday setting – sun, sea and sand – provides the key elements that damage your hair. For hair to be sleek and easy to style it must be well moisturized – a difficult task when you are exposed to extreme heat (and conversely extreme cold). A trip abroad is the perfect time to spend some money on good-quality hair products to protect, condition and bring out the best in your hairstyle.

rain

A sudden shower will always catch you unaware, so, unless you have an umbrella or hood to cover your hair and prevent it from getting soaked, dive into the nearest café and sit out the storm in comfort. The haircare rules for rain are similar to those for a humid climate: block out the excess moisture or pay the price. If you become drenched in a sudden downfall, only to watch the sun come out afterwards, be careful about letting your hair dry too quickly. The sun's rays will heat up the hair shaft, drying out the hair and causing it to lighten. You wouldn't try to blow-dry your hair when it is dripping wet – you would towel-dry it first and then rough-dry it before styling it properly – and the same care should be taken after a rainstorm. Carry a travel-sized bottle of conditioner in your beachbag or rucksack and if you get caught in a storm, smooth a little conditioner through your wet hair to help protect it while it dries naturally. Comb it through to leave it looking styled or tie it back loosely to look instantly groomed. If you have frizzy hair, smooth some anti-frizz serum through it, pull it back into a ponytail and let it dry naturally. When it's nearly dry, brush it straight, secure with hair grips and leave it until it is bone dry. You should be left with soft waves rather than corkscrew curls.

sea

Salt is your enemy here as it roughens up the surface of the hair, leaving it dull, damaged and porous. If your hair is colour-treated, the combination of sea salt and sun damage will make your colour fade rapidly. A leave-in conditioner (which contains UV protection) goes some way to protect the hair, as it coats the hair shaft and acts as a physical barrier to the salt. If you are happy to slick your hair back while you lie on the beach, use a sun-protection oil or wax on the hair to hold the cuticle down and prevent the hair shaft from being damaged. Always wash the salt out of your hair thoroughly at the end of each day.

chlorine

Chlorine is extremely bad for the hair, especially when combined with the sun's rays. When your hair is wet it acts like a sponge and is highly absorbent. So when you are in a swimming pool and wet your hair, chlorine enters the hair shaft, leaving it looking dull, dry and brittle. The best way to protect your hair is to wet it in the shower before heading for the pool and cover it liberally with a leave-in conditioner to coat the hair shaft, preferably one containing a UV filter to give extra protection from the sun's rays. Alternatively, try applying a non-water-soluble hair wax, which will act as an effective barrier (this is more suitable for shorter hair). Wash your hair thoroughly every day after swimming.

sand

Tie your hair back while you are on the beach as sand will roughen the surface of the hair. Give it a good, long rinse at the end of each day to get rid of any sand, then condition your hair, squeeze out excess moisture with a towel and gently comb it through.

wind

A cold, strong wind will cause some dryness. Keep your hair well conditioned and tie it back to keep it groomed and in place.

air travel

Ever gone on a long-haul flight and left the aeroplane with your hair glued to your scalp or crackling with static electricity? The air pressure in the cabin, coupled with the dry air, high altitude, nylon seat covers and magnetic field in the aeroplane causes even thick hair to become static. It's possibly the worst atmosphere for hair. Tie your hair back and place a silk headscarf over your headrest to minimize the static effect on your hair. Always travel with your hair free of styling products so that it can breathe. Take a small can of hairspray or a mineral-water atomizer in your hand luggage, plus a small comb or brush. Spritzing water over your head rehydrates and revitalizes your hair during a long-haul flight. Control static hair at the end of the flight by spraying a little hairspray onto your brush and brushing it through the hair to minimize flyaway strands (this will work just as well in cold weather when hair can also become static). Drink plenty of mineral water during the flight – it's important for your skin as well as your hair.

sun

The sun dehydrates the hair. The overlapping cuticles, which protect the centre of the hair shaft (its cortex), peel and break as they dry out in the heat. The cortex is made of keratin, a fibrous protein, which gives the hair its strength and elasticity. The sun's UV rays damage the hair by breaking down its protein structure. When the outer hair cuticle becomes damaged, or porous in the case of chemically treated hair, it's all the more easy for the sun's rays to enter the cortex causing dehydration and fading the hair colour. Sun exposure also increases free radical damage, causing premature ageing in your hair, just as in your skin. Look for products with built-in UV protection – everything from your conditioner to sun-protection spray for the hair. Or simply use regular sun-protection lotion on your scalp to prevent burning.

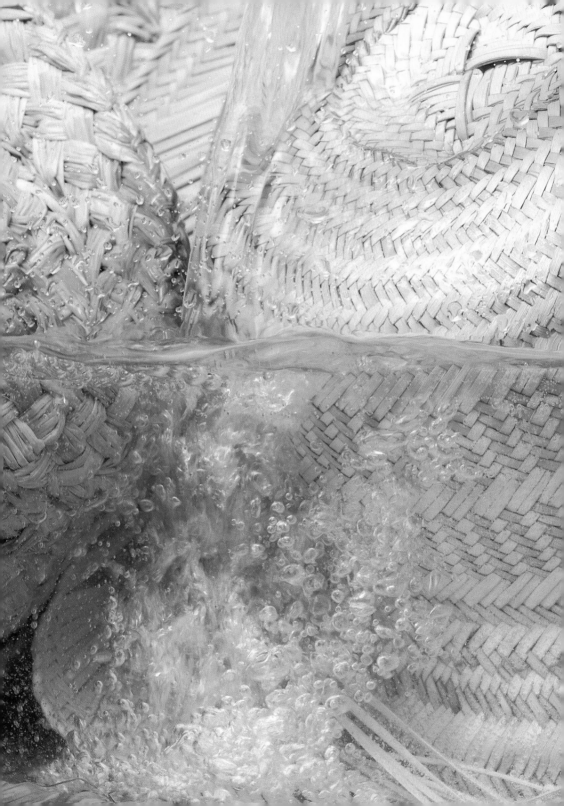

Dinner with Harry goes badly. Despite his recent lack of enthusiasm for their relationship, he's furious that Polly is calling it off. His male ego is taking a battering and he isn't going down silently. With his voice getting steadily louder, he argues through the main course and storms out before coffee arrives. Polly pays the bill quietly and goes home.

Waiting for her on her laptop is a message from Simon: 'Come away with me. Flights and hotel booked – leaving Saturday. Surprise destination. Pack for the sun.' Romance is exactly what Polly's been dreaming of, but sense tells her that this could be moving too fast. How can she take time off work? City deadlines are non-negotiable. More importantly, her highlights are in desperate need of attention – her natural colour's showing through and Polly, ever practical, has no intention of flying

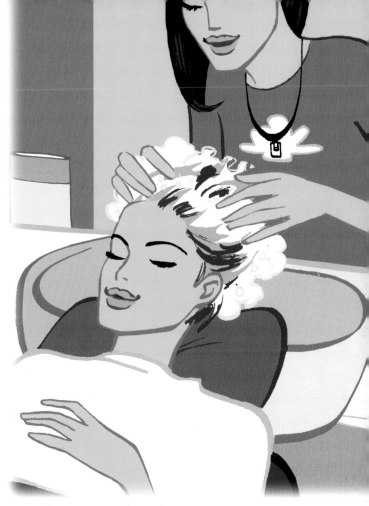

... polly's last-minute hair prep

off for a romantic week with a bad case of root regrowth. Her answer, she decides, will be governed by whether she can get a last-minute appointment with her colourist, Carolyn, before they're due to fly.

Next morning, Polly arrived at work early, determined to keep her mind off Harry (she does feel guilty for hurting him), and off Simon's exciting plans. The salon receptionist gives her an

appointment for a half-head of highlights and a hair mask. (It pays to be a regular customer.) Her decision has been made for her and, since she's taken so little of her annual leave, her boss is in no position to refuse her holiday request. Polly e-mails her reply to Simon: 'Great idea. See you at Heathrow. Can't wait.'

At the salon, Carolyn puts a few foils along Polly's parting and

around her hairline to even out the root regrowth. 'The sun will lighten your hair, Polly,' she says, 'so I'm not going to put too many highlights in now. Let's book you in for a cut and colour for your return and we can take a look at your hair colour then,' she advises. She also applies an extra-rich, creamy conditioning treatment to Polly's hair to give it a remoisturizing boost. Polly is now ready for her trip.

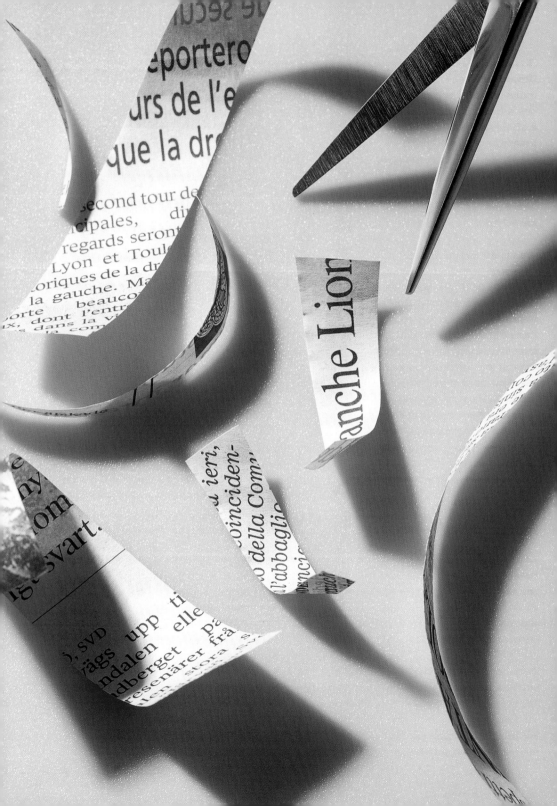

hair prep

In the run-up to your holiday, make time to book a consultation with your hairstylist and colourist to discuss your particular hair needs. Your salon can provide professional conditioning treatments that will keep your locks in top condition throughout your holiday and minimize the damage caused by various environmental aggressors while you are away. Ask your stylist to recommend an at-home intensive conditioning product and make a conditioning treatment part of your weekly haircare routine in the month before your holiday. This will give your hair a head start when it is faced with a change in climate.

Choose your haircare products carefully. Look for shampoos, conditioners and styling products that offer UV protection if you are going to be outdoors and in the sun on your trip. Make the most of the latest travel-sized versions of your favourite products – not only will they save valuable space in your luggage, they will also be convenient to carry around with you for on-the-go styling during the day. A great alternative is to decant your favourite products into small plastic travel bottles (available from good chemists) so you can travel light.

cut

A good haircut will compensate for a more casual holiday styling routine, so that you still look well groomed. Your hairstyle should be able to hold its shape even if you opt for minimal styling while you are away and dispense with the daily blow-drying, leaving your hair to dry naturally. Get your hair in shape by having a simple cut that requires only minimal effort to look good. A gently layered style, for example, will literally fall naturally into place and needs very little maintenance. Warn your hairstylist that you are going on holiday so that he or she can work your cut into an easy-to-manage shape and leave enough length to trim away any split ends on your return.

cutting considerations

Type of holiday If you are travelling in a hot climate or will be particularly active on holiday, you may want the option of wearing your hair up. Plan ahead – if your hair is short to medium length decide whether to let it grow longer so that it can be tied back.

Consult your hairstylist He or she might recommend having a few layers cut into your hair (to add shape) so that it looks good and is easy to style on holiday.

Be realistic You may want to inject some freshness into your look, so, as well as buying a few new holiday outfits, get advice from your stylist on different ways to style your haircut. Holidays are a great time for experimentation and trying out different products.

colour

Book a consultation with your colourist before your holiday. You may want to have your roots retouched or your colour revitalized with a tint so that it looks perfect for your trip. To look fabulous while you are away, have your hair colour done two to three weeks before you go, so that it is fresh and your hair has time to settle before your trip. However, depending on your destination and the climate there, your colourist may advise waiting for a full-colour treatment until your return. Blonde highlights will go even lighter in the sun, so warn your colourist if you are heading to the heat. It may be better to put a few tints around your parting and hairline, rather than using bleach on your hair before your trip. Similarly, lowlights and tints will fade in the sun, so your colourist might suggest a revitalizing colour treatment on your return, rather than before you go. Remember, chemically treated hair is porous and more vulnerable to the elements. If your hair is colour-treated or permed it will lose moisture faster than untreated hair and will need extra care while you are away.

blonde hair

Ask for a quarter-head of highlights rather than the full head of highlights before a trip to a sunny climate. This will colour the area around your face, on top of the crown and at the sides to refresh your colour. The sun will lighten your colour further while you are away. If you have lots of very light highlights through your hair, have a few natural blonde lights put through before your holiday as they will go lighter in the sun, so you will not damage the condition of the hair so much.

red hair

Have your colour done two to three weeks before your holiday and ask your colourist to mix a corresponding vegetable tint to take with you to refresh the red during your stay. Alternatively, use a coloured mousse (in the same shade as your hair) to refresh any light or brassy highlights. Test the colour on a white tissue before putting it on your hair, as some colours can be a bit misleading.

brown and dark hair

Ask your colourist to lighten a few tips of the hair around your face before a holiday to the sun. It looks naturally sunkissed and will lighten a little while you are away, leaving flattering highlights close to your skin.

colour considerations

1 Use a shampoo and conditioner formulated for colour-treated hair. You need moisturizing products that gently cleanse and condition the hair shaft. Deep-cleansing shampoos will lift colour tint out of the hair faster, so stick to gentle, daily formulas. Many shampoos and conditioners for colour-treated hair now contain UV protectants that can reduce sun damage.

2 You will always need a hair-colour treatment after your holiday, so if in doubt, wait until your return.

3 The ultimate protection for your hair colour is a hat or headscarf. Don't forget to tuck the ends of your hair into the hat as they are vulnerable to the sun if left exposed. The only way to avoid colour fading is to keep your hair out of the sun altogether.

hats for different face shapes

To properly protect your hair you need to keep it covered from the elements or out of the sun altogether. So wearing a hat is the most realistic option for shielding your hair while you are out and about. A baseball cap or headscarf will be better than nothing, as both cover your scalp and, to some extent, your hair. The best solution, though, is a hat with a decent brim that will shade your face and neck along with your hair. If you are sitting in the sun, always tuck the ends of your hair up into your hat – they are the driest part of your hair and the most vulnerable to damage from the environment.

oval faces

Virtually any hat shape will suit an oval face, as the proportions of the face are even. Choose one that you feel confident wearing, otherwise it will sit unused in your hotel room during your trip.

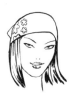

round faces

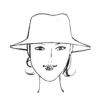

Balance a round face with a hat that has a good, high crown and a decent brim. A short crown and small brim will make your face look more round.

long faces

A hat that has a wide brim will offset the length of a long face. Choose one with a low crown – a high crown will make the face look even longer.

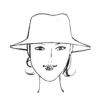

heart-shaped faces

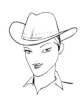

Most hats will suit a heart-shaped face, although a medium-sized brim (rather than a wide brim) will help to prevent the jaw line from looking too narrow.

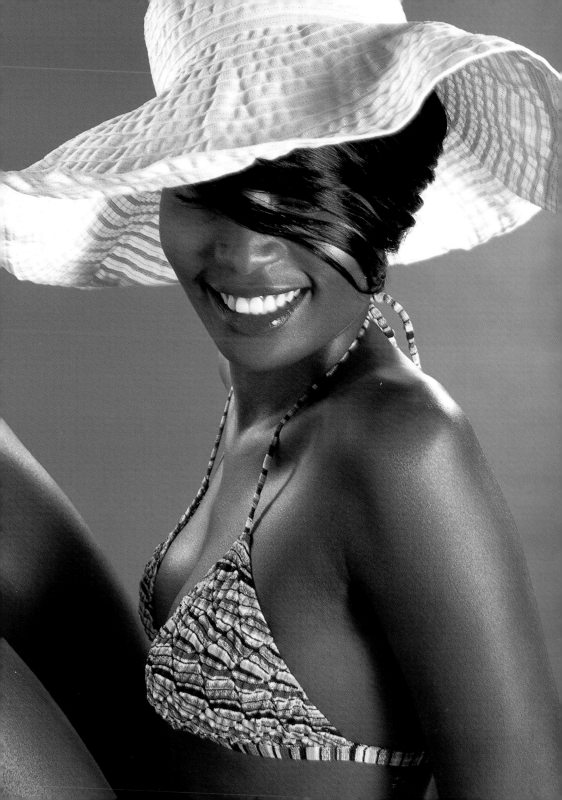

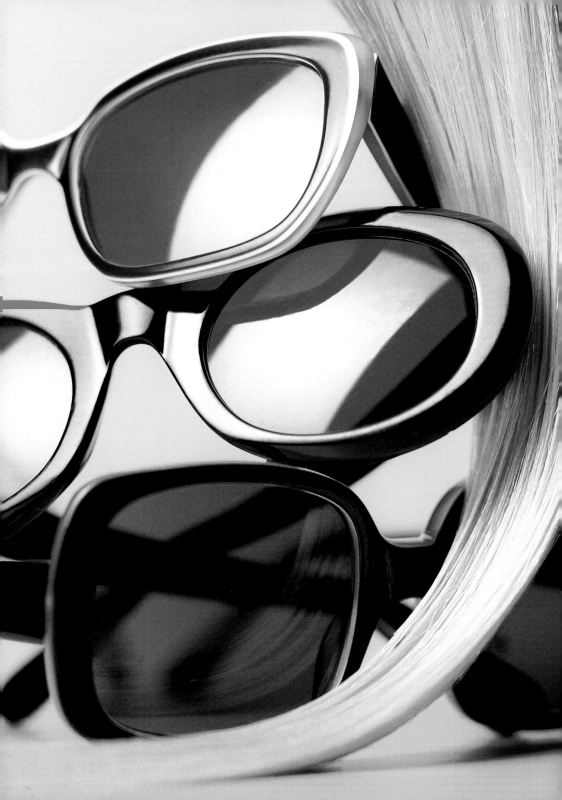

Back at the house after her interview at Aristo PR, Jaz is packing her overnight bag. Fashion PR guru, Astrid, has offered Jaz a job provided that she makes a good impression on a key client in Paris. They are catching the Eurostar train that evening and having dinner with one of Paris's top young designers. Tomorrow they have a meeting with a buyer at Galleries Marais department store to help the designer introduce

Jaz sprays some shine enhancer through her hair and brushes her thick, dark locks into a neat high ponytail. Then she smoothes down loose hairs with a natural-hold hairspray. She looks chic and ready for business. Jaz packs Kate's hair straightener. She knows she looks much more stylish with long, sleek hair and it usually has a natural kink when she wakes in the morning. Kate had reminded her that she'll find

complimentary shampoo in her hotel bathroom, so she just packs her own quick-rinse conditioner, as she hates using heavy conditioners on her hair. She finds a travel-sized bottle of mousse, which she pops into her washbag. It will help her to style her hair quickly in the morning. She also packs her multipurpose smoothing brush, which she can use when she blow-dries her hair.

... Jaz's trip to the fashion capital

his collection. Having spent months packing up clothes in the fashion department at *Gloss* magazine, Jaz is finally entering the fashion circuit for real. She has to perform well – and look directional and stylish for the next 24 hours.

Clothes are not a problem – she has Chrissie's wardrobe to choose from as well as her own. She decides to travel in black, low-slung trousers and take Chrissie's camel leather skirt and pointed, high-heeled boots, which look great with skirts and trousers. A couple of tops and her new knee-length military coat will cover all the options. What to pack for her hairstyling needs proves more of a problem. She's fairly certain the hotel will provide a hairdryer, but should she take hers in case? Jaz calls Kate to ask her advice. 'Why don't you borrow my hair straightener? Don't forget to pack a travel plug – a three-pin one won't work in Paris,' she says.

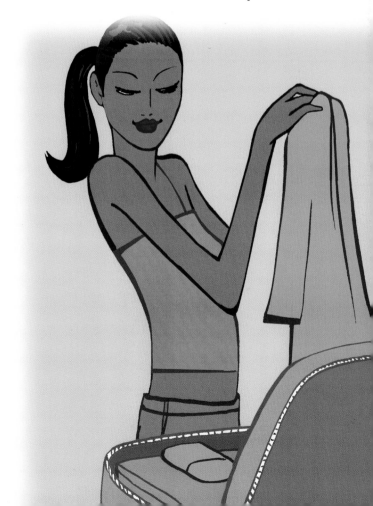

holiday hair tips

maintain the condition

Look after your hair on the plane – you don't want to damage it before you even get to your destination. Use a serum to protect it and spritz it with mineral water to rehydrate. Remember, salt water will dry and dehydrate the hair, so use a detox shampoo to cleanse away the salt and then condition with a moisture mask. If your hair does start to dry out, brush it every night with a natural-bristle brush. This will encourage natural oils, which will moisturize dry hair. While you are on holiday, remember to eat healthily and drink lots of water. Both your body and your hair will benefit.

protect, protect, protect

Ideally, wear a hat or headscarf to protect your hair from the sun's rays, but remember that heat can also damage the hair, so condition it well to prevent it from drying out. When you are not wearing a hat, make sure that you protect your scalp. It is part of your skin, so use sun-protection lotion to prevent it from burning.

special treatment for coloured hair

If you have coloured hair, seek advice from your stylist before you travel. You may need to have your colour done before or after your holiday, but either way it is very important that you get the right advice to achieve best results and maintain good condition. Delicate blonde hair will suffer if you spend lots of time in smoky clubs while you are away – serum will coat the hair shaft and act as a barrier, while detox shampoo will cleanse away any stains. If you have naturally brown hair that shows signs of fading in the sun, rinse beer through it to add depth and gloss, and then rinse well with water.

accessorize

Take a collection of coloured ribbons with you for dressing up your hair for going out. Ribbons make great accessories, are easy to pack and are available in lots of colours and materials that can be matched to any outfit. Hair fragrance is also very useful for freshening up the hair when you don't have time to wash it.

travel kit

brush and comb

A wide-toothed comb can be used on wet hair and is essential to banish holiday tangles. You should also pack a small all-purpose brush to cope with all your styling requirements.

hair accessories, grips and bands

Pack at least one stunning hair accessory for your holiday. If you're going to the sun, a tropical-flower clip would be ideal, whereas a diamanté comb or sparkly slides might be appropriate for a city jaunt. Matt hair grips are useful for pinning your hair up (in a twist or chignon), and covered elastic bands are the perfect quick-fix solution to most haircare problems – just tie your hair back. If you like to leave your hair loose, a wide fabric or zigzag headband is great for keeping it off your face.

products

If you're going on a beach holiday, take a gentle, everyday shampoo to wash the sun, sea and sand right out of your hair, while a detox shampoo is extra-cleansing for hair that is exposed to city grime or smoky clubs. A good conditioner with a UV filter is the key product for holiday hair. Don't expect to return with your hair in decent shape without it. In addition, pack an intensive hair mask for the ultimate moisture boost. Also essential if you are going to sunny climes is a sun-protection spray. As with suntan lotion, you should reapply this regularly throughout the day, especially after swimming.

travel plug

This is essential if you are heading abroad, since no hairdryer, straightener or electric curling tong will fit a foreign socket without it.

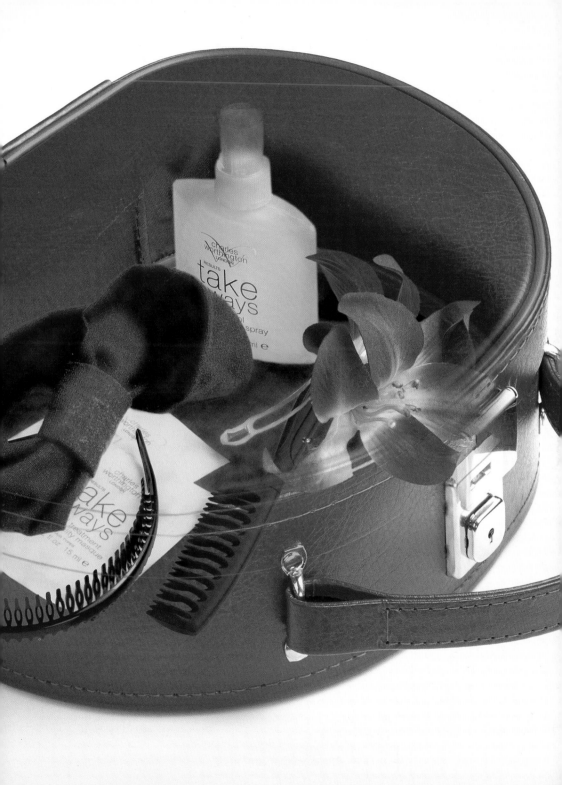

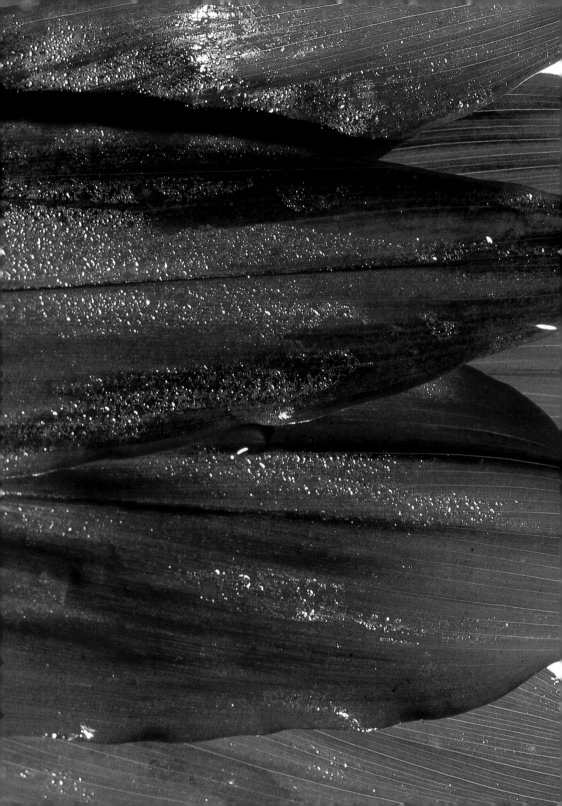

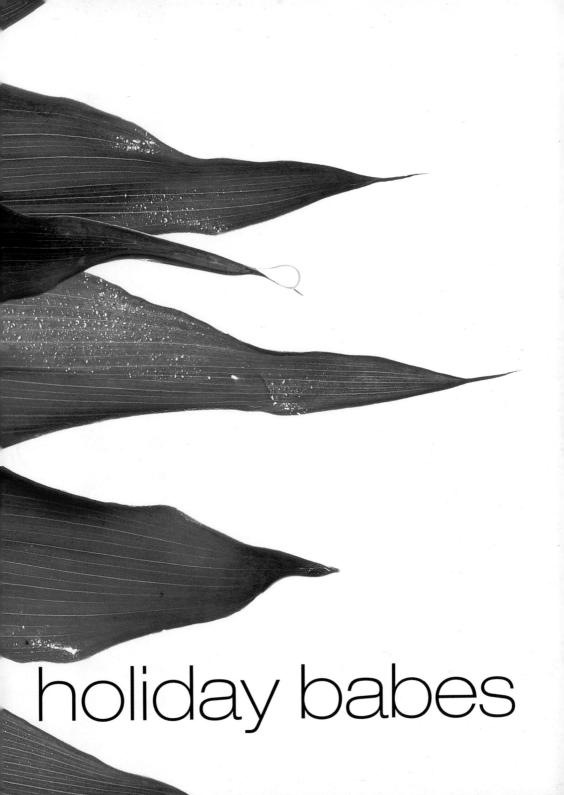

holiday babes

getting away from it all

Things were going from bad to worse in the marketing department at Crunch Biscuits. Matthew was too preoccupied with the latest Crunch Creams campaign to listen to Kate's idea for marketing the new low-fat biscuit. Kate found herself buried by a seemingly endless stream of marketing figures that she had to input into the system. Feeling demoralized, she opened her second pack of chocolate-chip cookies of the day and tucked in. Gazing around the office she saw all of her colleagues concentrating hard on their work. 'They're all so driven,' she thought to herself. 'And I'm stuck in this dead-end job with a boss who barely acknowledges me.' Picking up her bag, she quietly left the office and headed towards the nearest travel agent.

Five minutes later she was clutching an airline ticket. 'I'm suffocating in my life, and I'm going nowhere,' Kate thought. 'Polly's got her high-flying job in the City, Jaz's new job means she'll be surrounded by glamorous designers and fabulous-looking models, and Laura's working on a fascinating new real-life documentary.' The daily grind at Crunch Biscuits seemed mundane in comparison. 'I'm going to take charge of my life,' Kate resolved. 'A two-week yoga retreat in India is just what I need. I am going to relax and find my inner strength.' She walked slowly back to the office, sat down at her desk and filled out her holiday request form. Matthew barely read it as he signed it, and mumbled something about organizing adequate secretarial cover while she was away. Kate let his indifference wash over her – at last she had something to look forward to.

That evening at the house Jaz and Chrissie were in a restless mood. Polly's sitting room was covered with discarded fashion magazines, open CDs and the remnants of their supper. Laura was in her bedroom with the door closed yet again. She had been mooning around ever since the night in Cirque, was hardly talking to the girls and would rush to answer the telephone every time it rang. Jaz's trip to Paris had given her a taste for the high-life – she was in a full-on party mood. Chrissie was still smarting over her lack of success with Steve at Cirque. She was also a little concerned that her receptionist's job at Devastation Records was doing more to enhance her telephone skills than her career. She was still no closer to being 'discovered'. 'We need to get away, we need to get some sun,' Chrissie whined to Jaz. 'And how are we going to do that?' Jaz replied. 'We haven't got any money to spend on a night out, let alone a holiday.'

Chrissie knew it was true. Her uncontrollable shopping habit took care of any spare cash; she never could resist a new pair of shoes or the latest handbag. Jaz's unpaid work placement at *Gloss* magazine had cleared her savings account and her new job at Aristo PR put a considerable strain on her bank balance. She had been shopping every lunchtime since she'd started work, trying to put together a fashionable wardrobe for the office. 'Well, we do have our Visa cards,' said Chrissie, who had whipped hers out of her wallet and was waving it in the air. Jaz looked nervous. 'Do you think we should?' she said. 'You're only young once,' laughed Chrissie. 'Let's go and party in Ibiza. We can book it tomorrow.' 'You can book it on the Internet now,' said Laura, who had just walked into the room. 'I've just booked mine.' 'Your holiday?' shrieked Chrissie and Jaz together. 'Would you like to tell us where you're going?' demanded Jaz. 'And who with?' added Chrissie. 'The jungle in Sumatra, and John, as a matter of fact,' Laura replied coolly.

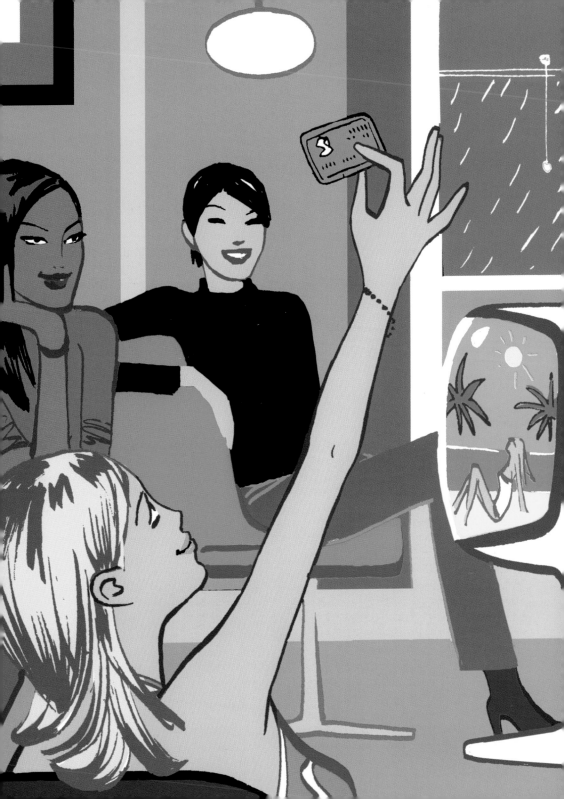

beach babe

There's not anything much you would rather be doing than lying on the beach and soaking up the rays. If you're not curled up on a sun lounger engrossed in the latest blockbusting romantic novel, you're strolling along the beach, taking a dip in the sea or enjoying some waterskiing or windsurfing when you have a burst of energy. You're a high-maintenance girl on the hair front: all that sun, sea and sand are going to make your hair drier than the Sahara Desert. That ice-filled cocktail from the beach bar won't help matters either.

hair solutions

Work water-resistant suntan lotion or a sun-protection hair product into the roots of your hair and spread it evenly across your scalp and around your hairline. Your head can easily be burnt through your hair by the sun and your hairline is a particularly sensitive area. If your scalp does get burnt, the hairline tends to peel first – which is not a great holiday look.

The best way to style your hair is to keep it simple during the day. Tie it back into a slick ponytail if your hair is long enough, or just comb it back once you've applied your sun protection through the roots if your hairstyle is shorter. Remember, though, wearing a hat is the best protection for your hair.

Make sure that you wash your hair thoroughly at the end of each day to rinse out all of the salt, sand and sun-protection product, then give your hair a good condition. If you have the time, apply your conditioner or hair mask and spend 20 minutes relaxing before rinsing to give the hair a real boost. Let your hair dry naturally if you're having a relaxed evening, or twist it up into a chignon if your hair is long enough for instant chic. Blasting your hair with a hairdryer or styling it with straighteners and curling tongs while you are in a hot climate is going to make dry ends worse – so try to limit your use of them to evenings when you want to look really special.

holiday tool kit

- Daily-wash shampoo
- Heavy-duty conditioner
- Nourishing hair mask
- Hair-protection spray with UV filter, or suntan lotion to use on your scalp
- Snag-free elastic hair bands
- Wide-toothed comb
- Headscarf or hat
- Styling product to suit your hair type

braid it

This is a fun, sexy look for beach parties and barbecues, but it is time-consuming to achieve and you need to set aside plenty of time to do it properly.

you need

Approximately 30 lengths of 5 mm (¼ inch) ribbon • sectioning comb • scissors for trimming ribbon

1 Starting at the front of the hairline, use a sectioning comb to neatly section off a piece of hair about 2.5 cm (1 inch) square.

2 Tie a length of ribbon securely around the section of hair at the roots.

3 Twist the section of hair all along its length, from the roots to the ends.

4 Tightly holding the ends of the twisted section of hair with one hand, wrap the ribbon neatly around the hair, crisscrossing as you go. Tie the ribbon securely around the ends of the hair and trim any excess to tidy.

5 Continue sectioning, twisting and braiding all over the head in the same way.

beach bunches

This is an easy style which you can do in no time at all before hitting the local nightspots. It's fun, cute and trendy – and perfect for clubbing, too.

you need

Sectioning comb • two snag-free bands • matt hair grips • glossing spray or light-hold hairspray

1 Use the comb to part the front section of the hair to one side. Then take the parting diagonally back to the opposite corner in the nape of the neck.

2 Comb the hair neatly into two ponytails and secure them with snag-free bands, making sure they are tight at the roots. Position the ponytails wherever you like, but for a quirky finish place them at different angles to each other.

3 Taking each ponytail in turn, twist the hair loosely and wind it around the base of the ponytail. Secure the ends of the hair into the ponytail base using matt hair grips.

4 Finish by lightly spraying the hair with a glossing spray or light-hold hairspray to hold down any stray ends.

mohican pony

Holidays are all about relaxing and having fun, so if you're feeling daring, let out the punk rocker in you and try this unusual style, which is guaranteed to turn heads wherever you go. You can either use coloured bands and cord or, as here, stick to neutral tones.

you need

Sectioning comb • snag-free bands • light wax • lengths of cord

1 Starting at the front of the head, take a section of hair from ear to ear, comb it up smoothly and tie it securely with a snag-free band.

2 Take the next section of hair, from above the ear on each side, comb it neatly to the top of the head and gather in the remainder of the last ponytail. Start to secure with the band as before, but this time leave the hair in a loop.

3 Repeat this process, working your way down the head to the nape of the neck. Leave the last section as a ponytail and smooth it with a light wax.

4 To finish, wind lengths of natural cord around the bands to disguise them.

HAIR SNIP

WHILE YOU ARE ON HOLIDAY, DON'T BE SCARED TO TRY OUT SOMETHING DIFFERENT WITH YOUR HAIR – REMEMBER, YOU PROBABLY WON'T EVER SEE THESE PEOPLE AGAIN. YOU CAN GET LOTS OF GREAT IDEAS FROM MAGAZINES

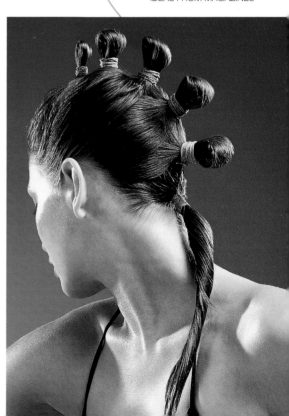

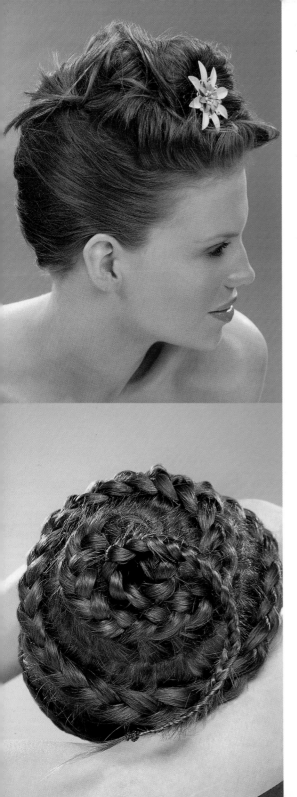

flower girl

Before you start, make sure the hair is free of any knots – you do not have to have clean hair for this style, but it will be more comfortable if you comb out any tangles.

you need

Sectioning comb • clip • matt hair grips • flower

1 Section off the top part of the hair and clip it temporarily out of the way, leaving the back hanging loose. Gently pull the sides and back section into a loose ponytail and twist it up to the crown, holding it in place with matt hair grips.

2 Unclip the top section and loosely twist it back randomly, securing it with matt grips.

3 Finally, add a fresh or fake flower and grip it in place.

french plait

You will probably need the help of a friend to do this and get the shape perfect, but once you have got it, it will probably last for a couple of days, and can be accessorized for the evening.

you need

Tail comb • snag-free band • hair grip • light-hold hairspray

1 Start by sectioning a 2.5 cm (1 inch) square piece of hair, parallel with one eye. Using a tail comb, start creating a spiral shape, running behind the ear towards the nape. While you are sectioning the hair, get your friend to start plaiting tightly against the scalp.

2 Carry on working towards the crown area, keeping an even spiral while doing so.

3 When all the hair is plaited, secure the ends using a band and secure the tail of the plait to the top section with a grip. Finally, use a little hairspray and the pointed end of the tail comb to push any flyaway hair into the plait to neaten.

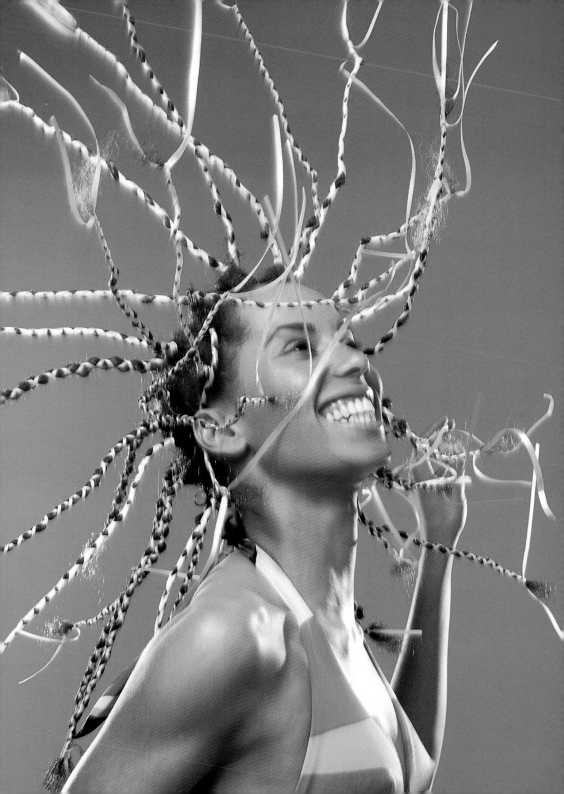

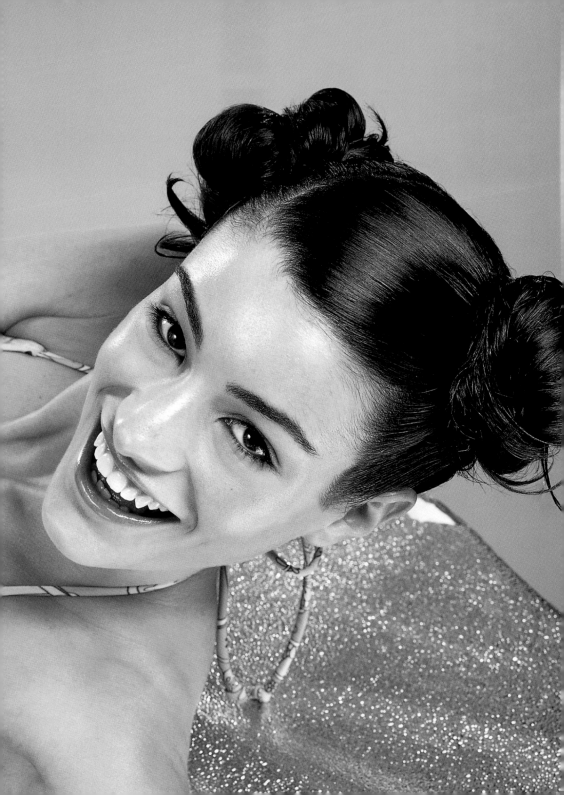

snow white

You can hardly wait to get to the mountains. During the day you keep your hair off your face with a warm hat or headband that covers your ears as you zoom down those mountain slopes. By night, you can be found enjoying the après ski in a dark, smoky bar.

hair solutions

The snow reflects the sun's rays, making them even more powerful, so protect your hair by using a good, leave-in conditioner with a UV filter. Keep your hairstyle simple, sporty and chic – glamour girls look out of place on the slopes. The cold makes your hair brittle and static, so keep a band or slide in your pocket to pin back flyaway hair.

holiday tool kit

- Daily-wash shampoo
- Leave-in conditioner (with UV filter)
- Snag-free elastic hair bands or hair slides
- Hair serum and hairspray (to help combat static)

ski chic

Poker-straight hair is the ultimate in sophisticated cool.

you need
Blow-drying spray • paddle brush • hairdryer • straightening irons • light water-based wax

1 Spritz the hair with blow-drying spray and use the brush to blow-dry it straight, section by section. Glide the hot straightening irons down the length of the hair.

2 Finish with a light wax for extra gloss.

ice queen

This style is a modern take on movie-star glamour. It's quirky yet sophisticated, and easier to achieve than it looks.

you need
Comb • large heated rollers • snag-free band • 2 hairnets (to match your hair) • hairpins • hairspray

1 Section your hair on large heated rollers to create volume and a good foundation to hold the style.

2 Section off the top rectangle of hair, from the crown to the temples, and sweep the remaining hair into a ponytail above the nape.

3 Backcomb the ponytail and cover it with a fine hairnet to form a bun. Secure with hairpins and hairspray.

4 Lightly backcomb the top section and twist it round, loosely. Secure the shape with pins and hairspray.

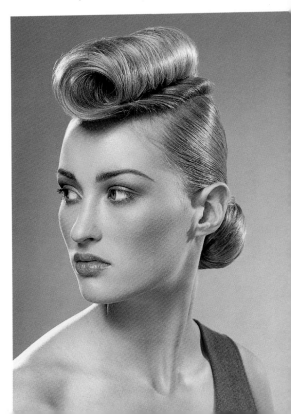

euro chick

Weekend city breaks are your thing. You like the stylish, cosmopolitan look with hair that will take you from chic boutique and café to museums and elegant restaurants.

hair solutions

The pollution and weather are your hair threats, so wash it daily with cleansing shampoo and condition it to put the moisture back in. Carry leave-in conditioner or serum with you in case you are caught in a rainstorm, and use sunglasses to hold hair off your face for a quick fix.

holiday tool kit

- Gentle cleansing shampoo
- Leave-in conditioner (with UV filter)
- Small can of hairspray
- Matt hair grips (to control stray hairs or pin hair up)
- Natural-bristle brush (to help keep hair free of dirt)
- Sunglasses (the stylish hair solution)

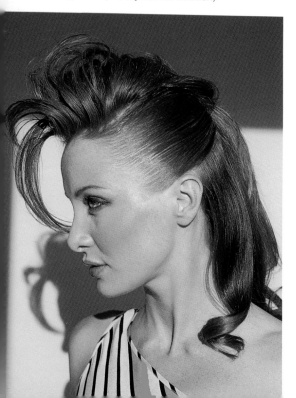

daytime sleek

This is the perfect style for city chic and can be easily adapted for a high-glamour evening look (see below).

you need

Comb • large heated rollers • flexi-hold hairspray • natural-bristle brush

1 Section the hair and wind it onto large heated rollers. The top section should go across to one side, the sides should go forwards and the back should go downwards.

2 Spritz with flexi-hold hairspray to give maximum hold and leave to cool.

3 Gently take the rollers out and smooth the hair using a bristle brush. If the hair is static, spray the brush with hairspray. Finish by spritzing with flexi-hold hairspray.

evening chic

Simply sweep back the sides and backcomb the top.

you need

Comb • large heated rollers • flexi-hold hairspray • natural-bristle brush • sectioning clip • firm-hold gel • matt hair grips

1 Prepare as for daytime sleek, above.

2 Clip the top section of hair out of the way and, using a firm-hold gel, comb the sides away from the face and secure with matt hair grips.

3 Backcomb the top section at the roots to give maximum lift and grip in place, letting the hair fall loosely over the face. Spritz with hairspray to finish.

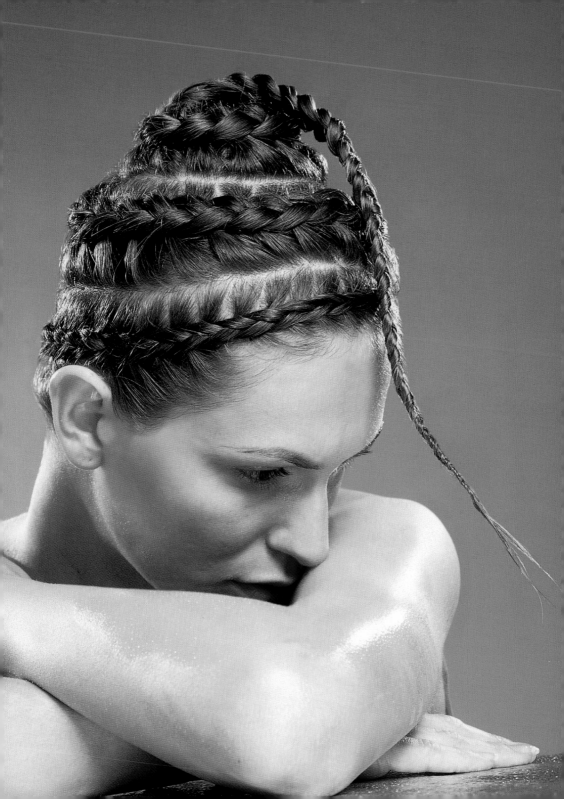

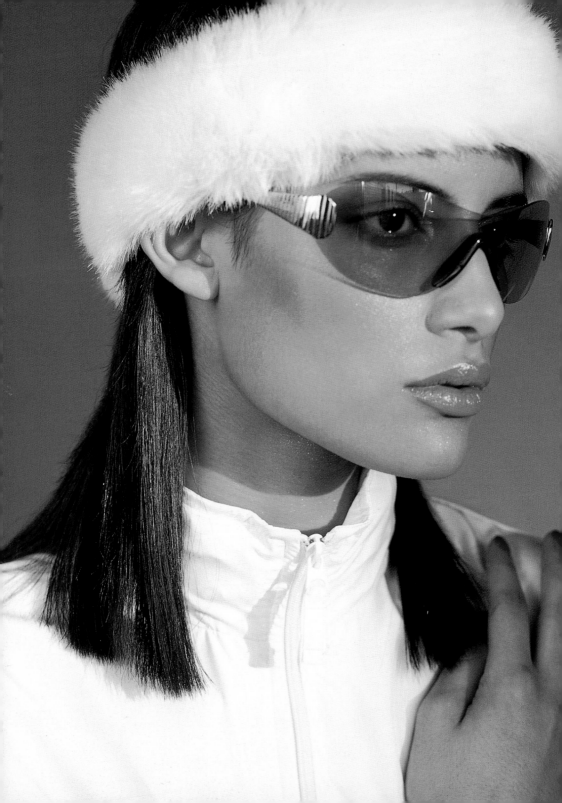

yoga fiend

Whether you're stretching your limbs in a yoga class or lying back for a massage, your hair is the last thing you should be worried about. Go for a natural look – creating big, glamorous hair is not a part of your holiday agenda.

hair solutions

Keep hair low maintenance by tying it back casually or letting it hang free. Pamper your hair as well as your body – apply a deep-conditioning mask, lie back and relax.

holiday tool kit

- Shampoo and conditioner
- Deep-conditioning hair mask
- Wide-toothed comb
- Snag-free elastic hair bands and hair slides

mask it

This is brilliant if you need to give your hair a treatment that will boost its moisture levels and combat dehydration.

you need

Comb • deep-conditioning treatment • snag-free band • fine hairpins • grips

1 Comb a moisturizing treatment through the hair, working right the way through the length, from the roots to the ends.

2 Twist the top section of hair loosely onto the top of the head, then pin it in place.

3 Secure the rest of the hair in a ponytail at the nape of the neck , and place a grip above and below the band.

hair treat

Even if your hair is in good condition, this treatment is ideal for keeping it out of the way while you pamper yourself.

you need

Comb • deep-conditioning treatment • snag-free bands • fine hairpins

1 Comb a moisturizing treatment through the hair as above.

2 Make a ponytail in the centre of the head and plait it, securing the ends with a band.

3 Wrap the plait around the head and secure it in place with fine hairpins.

HAIR SNIP

TAKE ADVANTAGE OF THE HEAT, WHETHER IT'S THE SUN OR A STEAM ROOM. HEAT ALLOWS THE TREATMENT TO PENETRATE DEEPER INTO THE HAIR SHAFT.

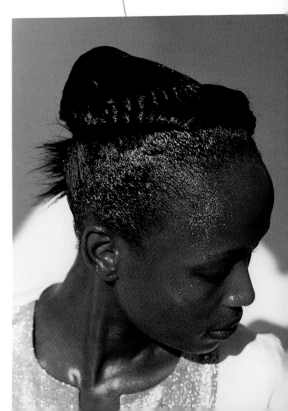

st tropez babe

When you are surrounded by celebrities, rock stars and royalty on holiday, you need a hairstyle that grabs some of the attention for you. Don't be afraid to make an impact with your hair. High-octane glamour is the only way to go – your hair has to be big, bold and full of body to make sure you really stand out from the crowd.

hair solutions

By day you need to look sleek and chic for lounging on the beach and hanging out in cafés drinking cappuccinos and watching the world go by. Stick to simple styles for low-maintenance elegance and remember, less is more for the daytime. Smooth ponytails, neat bobs and understated twists will give you effortless style. But by night, you need to rev up the pace with all-out glitz and glamour – go for big hair every time. The best way to achieve this look is by backcombing or backbrushing your hair, but remember only to backcomb the roots, otherwise you will be left with an uncontrollable bird's nest, instead of St Tropez glam! Remember, too, that all the sun and nightly hairstyling will take its toll on your hair. Whenever you get the chance on holiday, bathe your locks in a nutritious hair mask to keep the gloss and shine in your hair.

holiday tool kit

- Medium-hold setting spray and hairspray
- Medium-hold hair mousse
- Deep-conditioning hair mask
- Covered elastic hair bands
- Brush or comb for backbrushing

glamour curls

This hairstyle is truly 'big hair' like never before. The curls give great volume and texture, and the finger-styling creates a tousled, backcombed feel. This style works best if you have long hair, as the weight of your locks pulls the curls downwards.

you need

Medium-hold setting spray • hairdryer • heated rollers • medium-hold hairspray

1 Spritz medium-hold setting spray evenly through damp hair – the weather will determine how long this style will last, so be generous with the spray and make sure you cover the hair evenly. Then blow-dry your hair thoroughly.

2 Make sure your rollers are as hot as they can get. Then, starting at the top of your head, take medium-sized sections and wind them onto your hot rollers.

3 Spray the hair with medium-hold hairspray to help keep the humidity out. Leave the rollers to cool for as long as possible – use this time to put your make-up on and get dressed.

4 When the rollers are completely cool, gently take them out and apply some more medium-hold hairspray. Then, using your fingers like a comb, pull through the hair to break up the curls. (To make the style bigger, use your fingers to backcomb the hair.)

HAIR SNIP
ADD EXTRA BODY TO YOUR STYLE BY MASSAGING STRONG-HOLD HAIR MOUSSE TO THE ROOTS OF THE HAIR WHILE IT IS WET. FIRST, ROUGHLY BLOW-DRY THE HAIR TO REMOVE EXCESS WATER, THEN WORK THROUGH THE HAIR IN SECTIONS, LIFTING THE ROOTS UP AND AWAY FROM THE SCALP WITH A VOLUMIZING BRUSH TO GIVE EXTRA BODY TO THE HAIR AS IT DRIES.

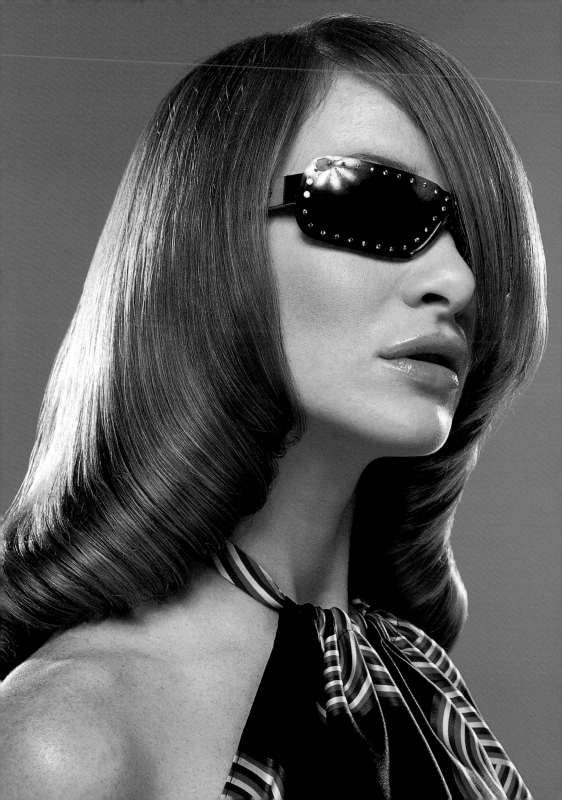

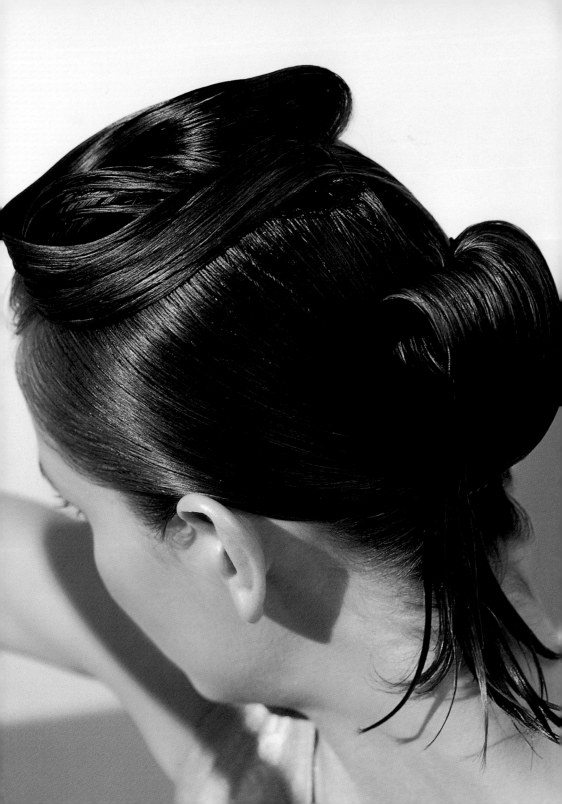

va-va-voom

A less curly – but equally glam – version of big, big hair. This is pure rock-chick-meets-European-princess.

you need

Hairdryer with diffuser • blow-drying primer • blow-drying spray • large velcro rollers • hairspray • natural-bristle brush • light shine spray

1 Start by blow-drying the hair using a blow-drying primer to give body and 'guts'.

2 When the hair is 90 per cent dry, spritz it evenly with blow-drying spray.

3 Using large velcro rollers, wind medium-sized sections of hair straight down onto the base of each section. Make sure that you wind the hair in the desired direction, otherwise it will be difficult to style.

4 Dry the hair using either a portable hood dryer or a diffuser. Make sure the hair is 100 per cent dry, then let it cool right down.

5 Starting at the bottom and working up, take out the rollers, making sure that you do not tangle the hair.

6 Spray the hair with hairspray, then gently backbrush the root area to create lift.

7 Finish by smoothing a bristle brush over the surface of the hair and spray using a light shine spray.

accessorize it

The severity of this sleek style is counteracted by the pretty hair grips, which add instant sexiness and softness.

you need

Hairdryer • light-hold mousse • paddle brush • straightening irons • blow-drying spray • pretty hair grips • wax

HAIR SNIP
TAKE A HAIRPIECE AWAY WITH YOU TO ADD INSTANT LENGTH AND VOLUME TO YOUR LOCKS. THIS CAN BE ATTACHED AT THE BACK OF THE HEAD TO GIVE THE ILLUSION OF LENGTH, AND THE JOIN CAN EASILY BE DISGUISED WITH YOUR CHOSEN ACCESSORIES.

1 Start by blow-drying the hair smooth using a light-hold mousse and a paddle brush.

2 Starting at the nape, straighten the hair section by section using the straightening irons. Spritz each section with blow-drying spray first to protect the hair.

3 Tuck the front sections behind the ear and hold them in place with your chosen accessories.

4 Finish the ends with wax to add texture.

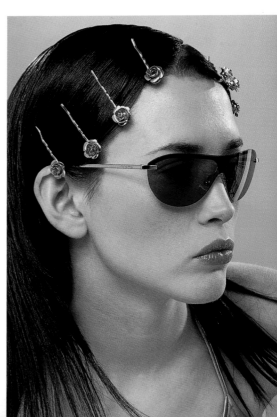

The pressure of keeping their relationship quiet at work, along with the normal demands of a fast-paced job in TV, has made Laura and John decide to take a break. They are both passionate about wildlife and quickly agree on a ten-day trek in the jungles of Sumatra to see orang-utan in their natural habitat. It's far from a comfort holiday but they both know they'll come back having had an adventure. Laura looks at the clothes and toiletries laid out on her bed and sighs as she lifts up her compact rucksack. Despite her tomboy attitude she can't seem to organize her belongings into vital, possible and unnecessary items. It's early days in her relationship with John and while she won't need kitten heels or a hairdryer, she wants to look attractive and effortlessly cool. She'll be carrying her rucksack from one camp to the next, so she needs to make sure it's as light as possible. A washbag full of products is a definite no: it seems to weigh a ton. She gets tough and singles out four T-shirts, two pairs of shorts, a swimsuit, trekking boots and

... laura's hair-raising dilemma

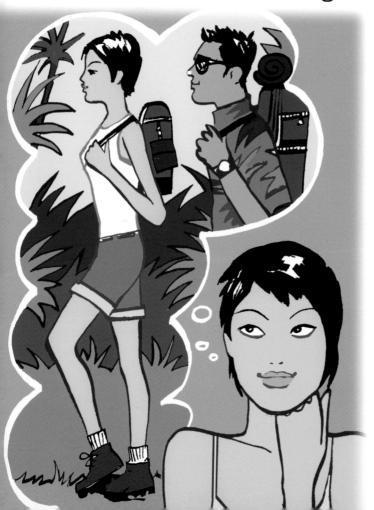

sandals. She faces the question of cosmetics. A light, frequent-wash shampoo and leave-in conditioner with UV protection are a must. She'll be lucky to find a bucket of water to wash with along the trail and she needs to protect her hair from the damaging rays of the sun. Her cropped hair will dry quickly in the heat, but the humidity will play havoc with her hair and she doesn't want to face John with a bad case of cotton-wool hair. A small bottle of anti-frizz serum should do the trick – she can use it sparingly to give texture to her hair, weigh it down a little, hold her style and stop the ends from frizzing. Suntan lotion, after-sun cream with insect repellent, mascara, toothpaste, a tooth-brush and an all-over face and body cleanser all make it into her washbag. A wide-toothed comb will help keep tangled hair at bay. She's managed to halve her packing in one go.

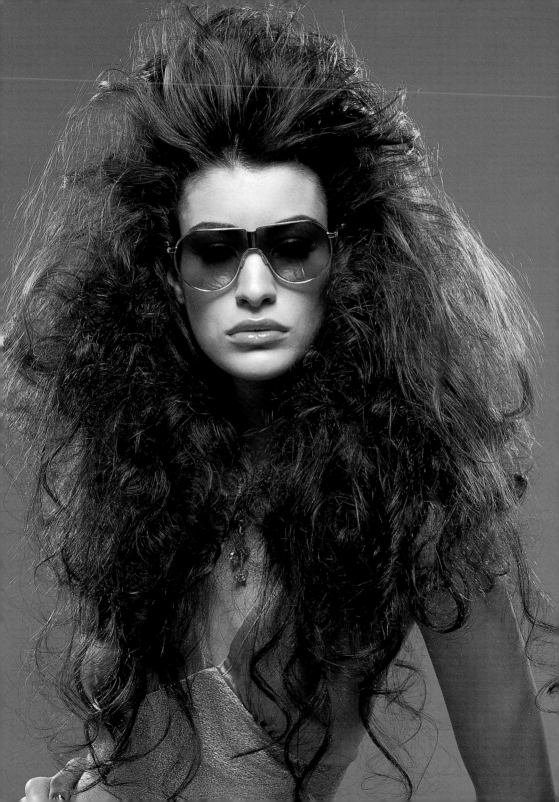

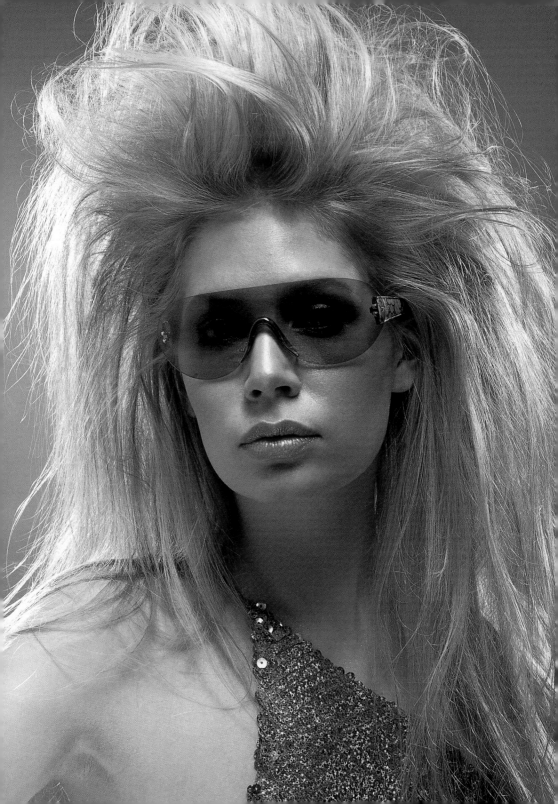

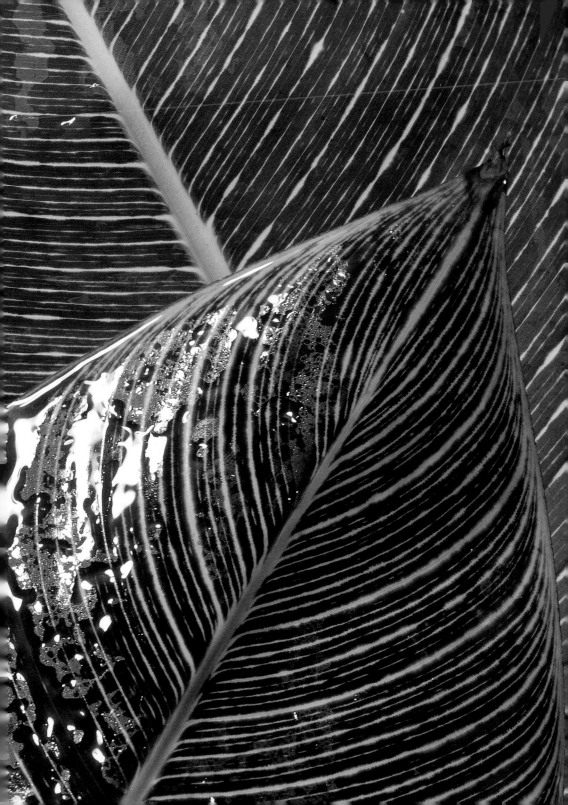

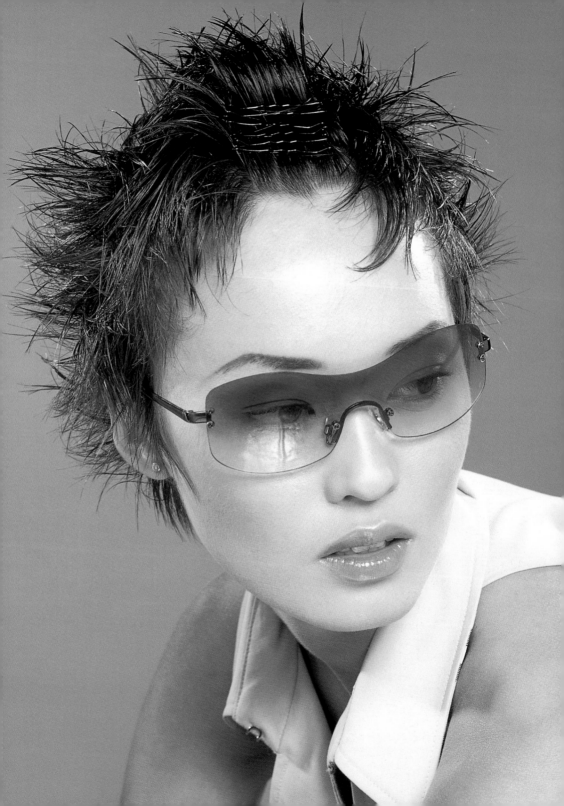

backpack girl

Freedom is a rucksack on your back and a guidebook in your hand. Your holiday is far from luxurious, but whether you're trekking in a jungle or camping on a beach, you'll be having the time of your life. You have to carry your bag on your back, so everything you pack must be useful.

hair solution

Take away your favourite products in travel sizes to cut down on space and weight. You need a gentle, daily shampoo to rinse your hair quickly – your bathroom facilities will probably be basic. Use a leave-in conditioner to protect your hair from the sun. Take only the styling products you'll need to create a low-maintenance, casual look. Hair serums will help prevent frizz if you're in a humid climate and the easiest quick fix will be to tie your hair back. Slides and accessories will give instant glamour.

holiday tool kit

- Gentle daily-wash shampoo
- Leave-in conditioner (with UV filter)
- Hair serum and hair wax (to perk up a short hairstyle)
- SOS glamour kit: hair grips, accessories and snag-free elastic hair bands

short 'n' sweet

You do need a textured haircut to create this funky style, but it's easy to maintain when you don't have much time.

you need

Hairdryer • light gel spray • firm-hold wax • hair grips

1 Dry your hair using a light gel spray to give lift at the roots.

2 When your hair is dry, mould it into shape, then work in a firm-hold wax to create texture.

3 Comb the fringe (bangs) back from the face and secure it with hair grips.

dreadlocks

Dreadlocks look cool but they can be difficult to comb out, so be certain you like the look before you commit.

you need

Fine-toothed comb • light-hold hairspray • wax

1 Take a 2.5 cm (1 inch) section of hair and gently twist it from roots to ends, then spritz it with light-hold hairspray.

2 Using a fine-toothed comb, gently backcomb along the length of the hair.

3 Run wax over the surface of the dreadlock to prevent it from unravelling.

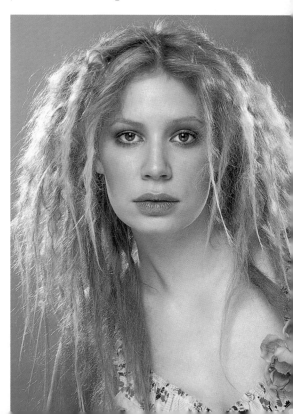

fresh-air queen

Whether you're walking, mountain biking or horse riding through the hills, your ideal holiday is always in the countryside. Glamour is not top of your list, but practicality is key for your activities. In the evenings you go for a natural look, making the most of your hair with an easy-to-style cut that holds its shape with minimum effort.

hair solutions

Depending on your destination, you're likely to be exposed to sun, wind or rain all day, so protect your hair with a leave-in conditioner. Keeping your hair out of the way will be essential. Use styling wax or an extra-hold gel on short hair to work it back from the face and tie longer hair back. A little hairspray will hold down those loose strands. Gently style your hair in the evenings with the help of a mousse – it'll make your post-shampoo styling quicker and help hold your hairstyle for longer.

holiday tool kit

- Daily-wash shampoo
- Leave-in conditioner (with UV filter)
- Wax, styling gel or mousse and hairspray
- Snag-free bands or grips (to keep hair under control)
- Wide-toothed comb (to keep tangles at bay)

country curls

Just wear plaits by day and unravel them for evening curls.

you need

Comb • styling spray • snag-free bands • clip

1 First shampoo and towel-dry your hair; then comb out any tangles and spritz with styling spray.

2 Section the hair into 5 cm (2 inch) square sections and plait them tightly from roots to ends. Fasten with bands and dry the hair in the sun or with a hairdryer, then unravel the plaits. Clip up the top section of the hair and add a flower.

twist and shout

These easy-to-do twists create a relaxed, fresh look.

you need

Hairdryer • blow-drying primer • hairpins • wax

1 Dry the hair using a blow-drying primer spray for extra lift and hold. Twist the top section of hair onto your crown and secure it with pins, letting strands fall out for added texture.

2 Twist the back section up and pin it as before, again leaving strands to fan out.

3 Finish by using wax on the ends to add definition.

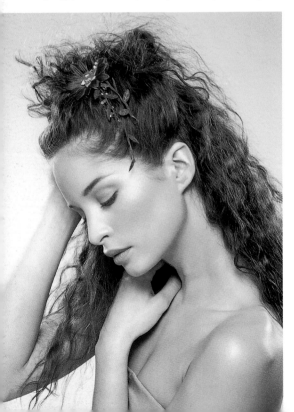

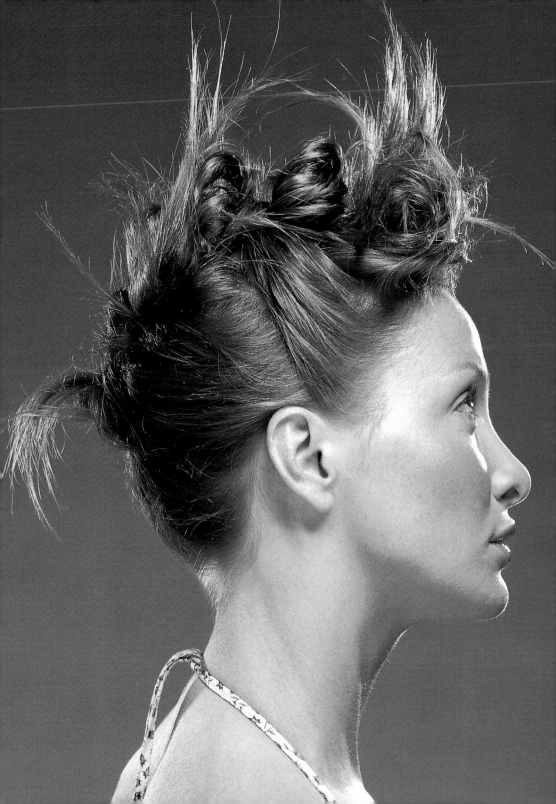

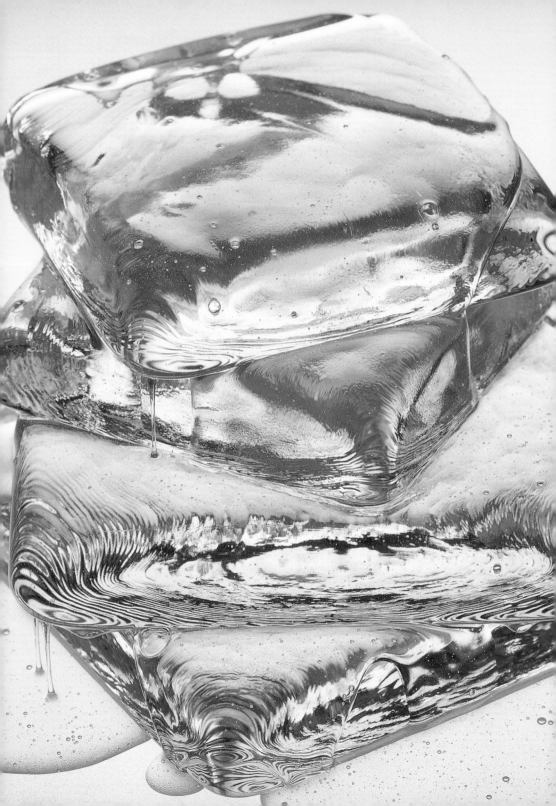

Chrissie and Jaz stumble onto the beach, hiding the signs of their hangovers behind dark sunglasses. Having clubbed through the night until 6 am, they haven't had much sleep and they hardly have the energy to do more than put on their bikinis and walk the short distance from their beds to the beach. They spot two free sun loungers and, with a sudden burst of energy, run down the beach to grab them.

Jaz and Chrissie are having a fantastic time. The night before they'd made an extra effort to show off their newly acquired golden tans by wearing matching micro miniskirts and sparkly lycra tops which they'd bought specially for their holiday. (They knew they'd attract more attention if they wore identical outfits.) Jaz had decided to straighten her hair to a glossy sheen by spritzing on some anti-frizz serum and carefully running the straightening irons along each section from the roots to the ends. She'd then pulled back the top and secured it with a sparkly diamanté clip. Chrissie had scraped her hair back into a high ponytail and secured a platinum-blonde hairpiece to its base, covering the join with a strand of her own hair. The length of hair down her back almost reached her waist and she looked fantastic. 'Aren't you ready yet?' she'd called to Jaz, 'We've got some partying to do!'

Chrissie and Jaz party on ...

'That's me done for the day,' laughs Chrissie, as she spreads her towel across the lounger, flops down and closes her eyes. Jaz quietly begins her daily ritual of sun protection. She smoothes suntan lotion all over her body and then squeezes a blob of leave-in hair conditioner onto the palm of her hand and mixes some suntan lotion into it. She works the mixture over her scalp and around her hairline. 'You are ridiculous Jaz,' teases Chrissie. 'I can't believe you bother doing that every morning.' 'Just protecting myself from the sun,' replies Jaz, as she combs her hair back into a loose ponytail. 'You ought to wear a hat, with your blonde hair and fair skin,' she warns, uncharacteristically sensible. 'This holiday is about being wild and crazy, Jaz,' says Chrissie. 'I don't remember you playing it safe last night ...'

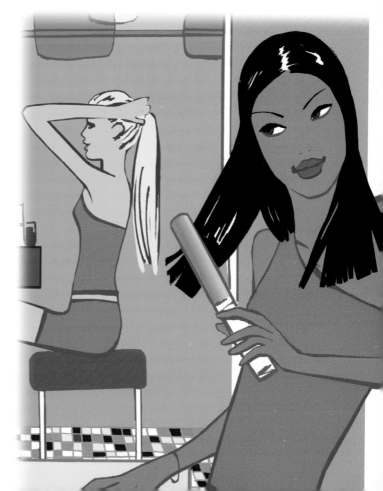

club bunnie

From Ibiza to Aya Napa, you can be found dancing the night away from dusk until dawn and then sleeping off your hangover in the sun by day. This type of holiday is really going to put your hair to the test. You'll be exposing it to the sun's rays during the day and smoky environments by night. And not only that – you'll also be subjecting it to heavy-duty styling to create glamorous looks with a high wow-factor.

hair solutions

As well as giving your hair a daily cleanse and detox, you also need to condition it on a daily basis to keep it from drying out during your high hair-maintenance holiday. Your focus is going to be on creating sassy, funky styles for the evening, so make sure you pack your favourite strong-hold styling products to give extra staying power to your hairstyle. A rich, conditioning hair mask will help to keep your hair moisturized, so that you don't return home with dried-out, stressed tresses – use it at least twice a week on your trip.

holiday tool kit

- Detox shampoo
- Leave-in conditioner (with UV filter)
- Hair mask
- Extra-hold styling products: mousse, hairspray, wax and serum (depending on your hairstyle)
- Selection of pins and grips for stylish updos
- Snag-free bands (for beach hair during the day)
- Glitzy hair accessories for instant glamour, such as flowers, butterflies, feathers and gemstones

funky hair

Funky hair is what every club bunnie needs. The idea is to look hip, sexy and effortlessly cool. This dishevelled look is easiest to create on short and medium-length layered styles. You just need plenty of firm-hold mousse to make sure your style lasts as long as you do.

you need

Firm-hold mousse • hairdryer (with diffuser) • several plastic hair combs • glossing spray

1 Generously apply firm-hold mousse, making sure all the hair is completely covered.

2 Gently blow-dry the hair until it is 80 per cent dry using a diffuser or the slow setting on your hairdryer.

3 When the hair is 80 per cent dry, place combs firmly into the hair as needed, positioning them so that the hair fans out in different directions.

4 Once you are happy with the shape your hair is creating, continue drying your hair until it is completely dry; this will ensure your hair stays up all night.

5 Finish with a good spritz of glossing spray, which will make your hair extra shiny.

tips for club bunnies

Use lots of products to give your hair substance and hold – there is nothing worse than a collapsed hairdo halfway through the night.

Use snag-free bands and matt hair grips – these will hold the hair in place without damaging it.

If you have very long or thick hair, try to keep it tied back. This will keep you cool and prevent your hair from getting sweaty and collapsing when you're dancing.

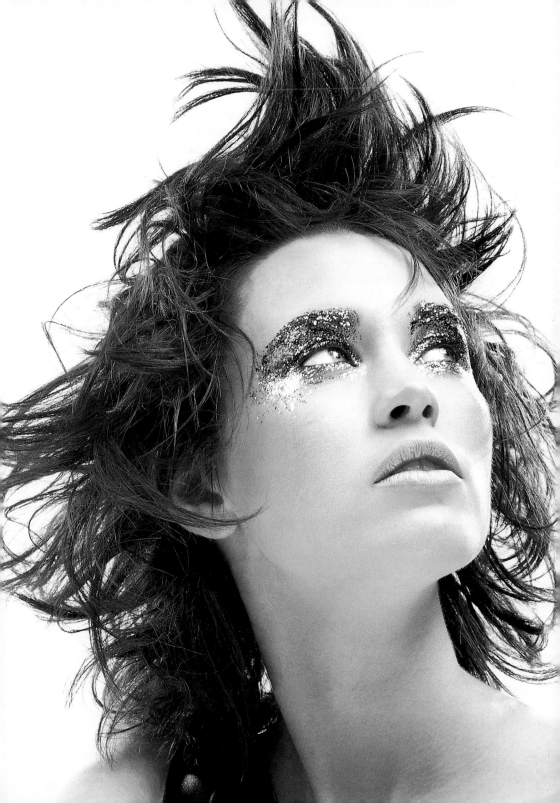

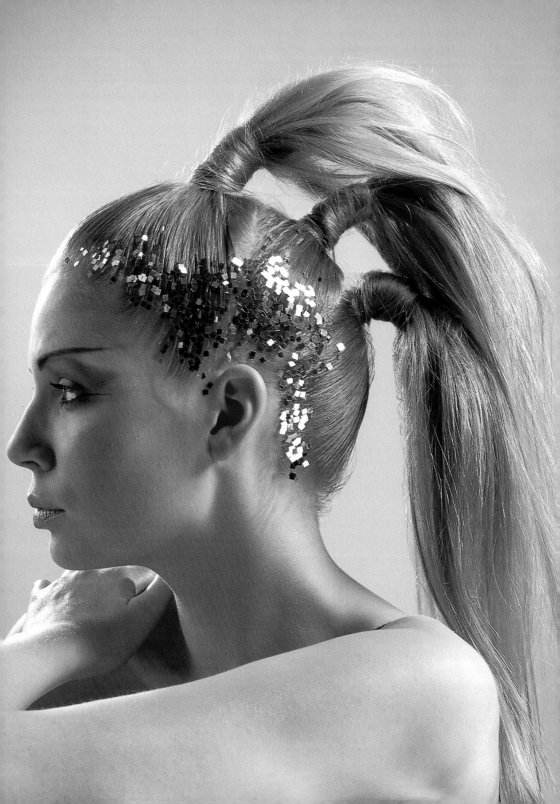

high pony

This is a sleek, high-glamour look that will look great and help keep you cool when you are dancing.

you need

Hairdryer • light-hold mousse • paddle brush • straightening irons • comb • 3 snag-free bands • hairpins • glitter and gel (optional)

1 Blow-dry the hair smooth using light-hold mousse and a paddle brush. Then straighten the hair section by section using the straightening irons.

2 Divide the hair into three horizontal sections, securing each with a snag-free band. Then wrap a strand of hair around the base of each bunch to disguise the band and secure it with hairpins.

3 Backcomb the base of each ponytail to make it stand away from the head and, for extra drama, use gel to stick chunky glitter along one side of the head.

chopstick twists

This excellent hairstyle is great for a big night out, and surprisingly quick to achieve (see overleaf).

you need

Hair grips • firm-hold hairspray • chopsticks

1 Taking a 2.5 cm (1 inch) square section of hair, twist it tightly from ends to roots, letting the hair wind down on itself.

2 Wind the ends of the hair tightly around the base and secure it with a hair grip.

3 Continue by winding sections of hair all over. When you have twisted all the sections, apply firm-hold hairspray.

4 Accessorize the twists with chopsticks (as shown here), or with flowers, feathers or beads.

ponytail tips

Make sure ponytails are firmly secured to prevent them from slipping or loosening. Hold them in place with snag-free bands or wet string, which contracts as it dries, holding the hair even more tightly.

To give a neat, slick finish, wrap a section of hair around the ponytail base to cover and disguise the hair band. Secure the section of hair in place using a matt hair grip.

Use chunky glitter to accessorize your hairstyle. This can be fixed in place by applying a strong-hold gel to the desired area before adding the glitter. Finish with a strong-hold non-aerosol hairspray.

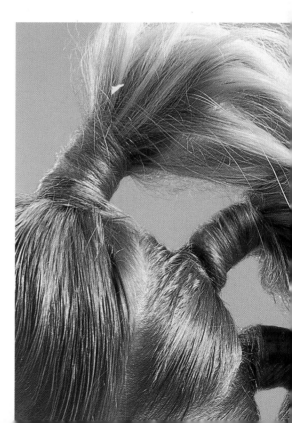

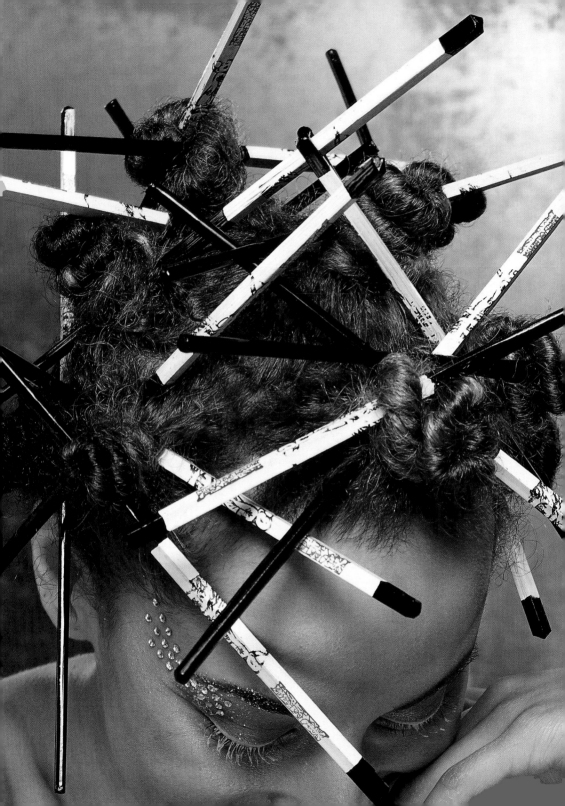

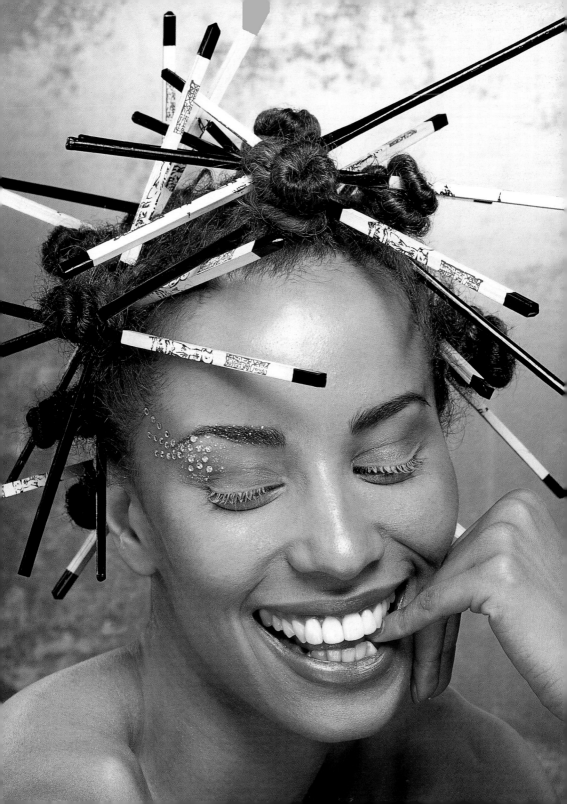

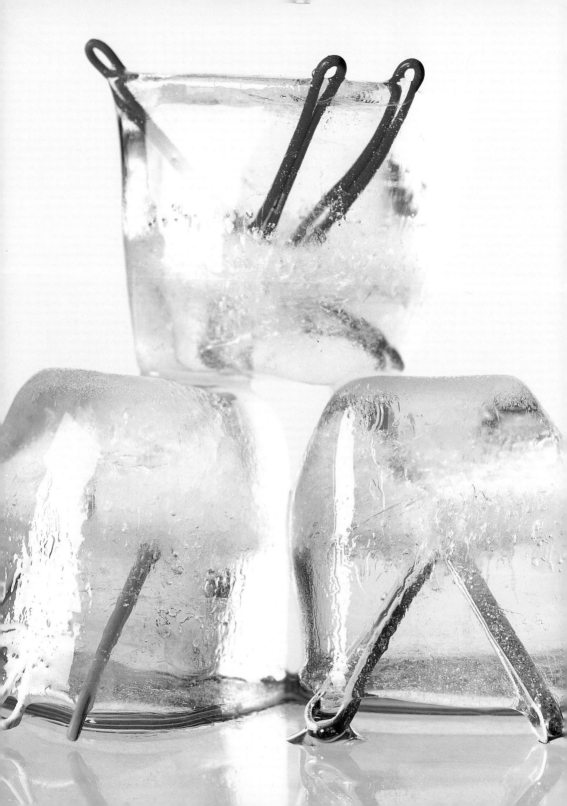

holiday hair
quick fixes

1 Take a bottle of fresh tap water with you to the beach to rinse the sea salt out of your hair throughout the day. Remember to do this, and then to reapply leave-in conditioner (with a UV filter) or sun-protection spray to your hair (and suntan lotion to your face and body) after every dip in the sea.

2 Keep a travel-sized bottle of leave-in conditioner or a travel-sized can of hairspray in your backpack or beach bag at all times in case of emergencies. You can use either one of these products to seal the ends of your hair or slick down stray ends for a quick style fix.

3 Keep a thick, cotton-covered hair band handy to tie back your hair for on-the-spot grooming. As an extra precaution, smooth a little conditioner over the band to help prevent you from snagging or tearing your hair when you remove it later on.

4 This is a great quick fix for naturally curly hair. After washing your hair as normal, apply a firm-hold styling mousse evenly through your hair. Taking one small section of hair at a time, twist each one from the roots to the ends. Carry on until your whole head is covered in twists of hair. Then dry it slowly using a diffuser on your hairdryer, being careful not to disturb the twists of hair while you dry them. When your hair is dry, unwind the twists and you'll be left with a head full of spiral locks.

5 Apply hair-protection lotion as often as you would apply your regular sunscreen to your face and body. The golden rule is to reapply. One spritz in the morning does not give day-long protection.

6 If it all gets too much, simply push your hair back from your face and hold it in place with your sunglasses. Wearing your sunglasses as if they were a hair band is a stylish – and fail-safe – quick fix.

7 If you have short hair, take styling wax with you on holiday. You can use it to rework your hairstyle into funky chunks in an instant if you get caught in the rain or are suffering the consequences of a humid climate.

8 Tie back long hair at the nape of your neck, rather than scrunching it up on the top of your head while you are out and about. This way you will avoid exposing the ends of your hair to the sun (important even on a cloudy day when the UV rays will still be strong), thereby preventing them from becoming dry and brittle.

9 Sun-protection body lotions and oils can be used on your hair (in small amounts only) to protect your scalp from the sun. Apply a few drops through your hair and work it onto your scalp by massaging with your fingertips. Don't forget to apply sun protection to your ears, as they will be exposed to the sun, especially if you tie your hair back.

10 Give yourself a cool sporty look and slick back those loose ends with a wet-look sun-protection gel containing a UV filter (go for the no-hold type). This will give your hair extra protection if you are swimming and sunbathing a lot; it works well on long hair if it is being tied back, as well as on short hair, and can be reapplied regularly during the day to keep the sun-protection factor up.

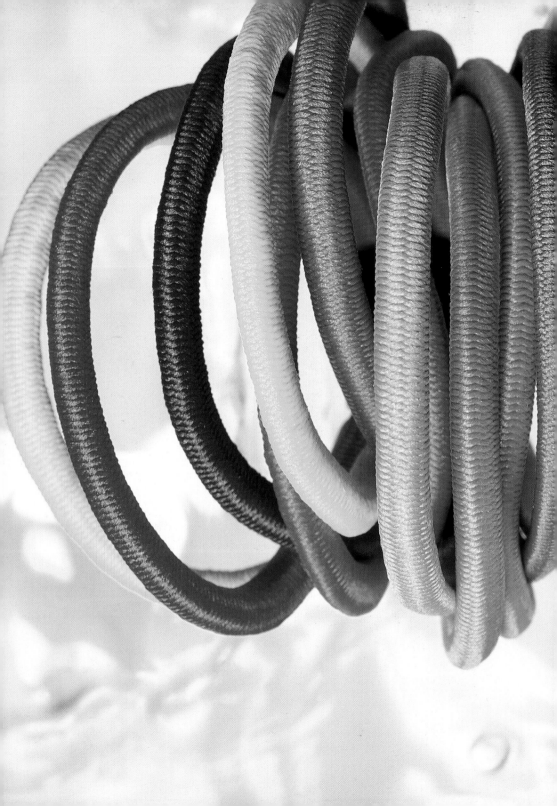

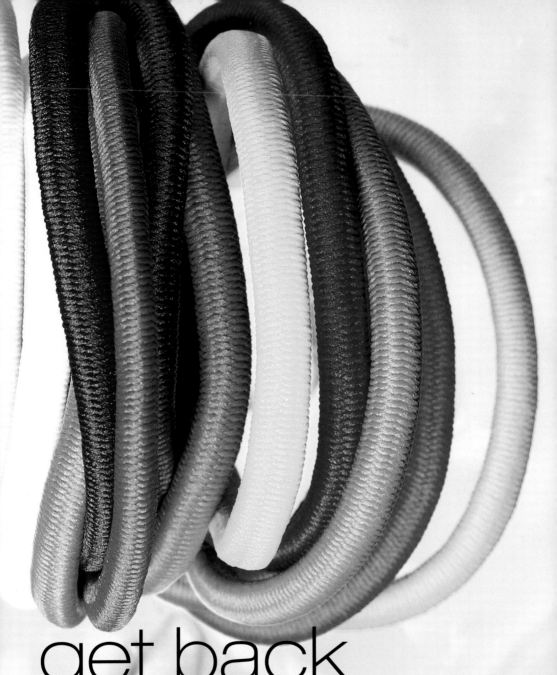

get back
into shape

exotic experiences

On her third morning, Kate woke in her tiny room at the ashram in Kerala. It was only 6 am and yet she felt completely awake and healthier than she had in ages. Her daily routine of yoga classes, meditation and cleansing Ayurvedic treatments were doing the trick. She felt more confident about herself. Her vegetarian diet and daily exercise regime had given her that sought-after smooth stomach. She knew she looked good, despite the fact that she hadn't bothered to put on even a stroke of mascara since she'd arrived. The only thing that didn't agree with the Indian climate was her hair: it had frizzed into bouncy ringlets and there was little Kate could do about it. She surprised herself by not caring in the least.

Stretching happily, Kate jumped out of bed and threw on some linen drawstring trousers and a white, fitted T-shirt. She grabbed a towel, slipped on her flip-flops and set off for her morning yoga lesson. 'Good morning,' said a voice behind her. It was Luke, a tall, suntanned guy who was living at the ashram for six months' training to become a yoga teacher. 'Did you sleep well?' he asked Kate. 'Fantastically,' she replied. 'I haven't felt this rested in ages. I won't know myself after two weeks here.' 'I thought I'd join your class this morning,' said Luke. 'Great,' said Kate, trying to contain her delight. She hadn't met anyone like Luke before; he was calm, intelligent and genuine to everyone he met. She was fascinated to find out more about him, what had drawn him to the ashram and why he wanted to become a yoga teacher. Perhaps breakfast after their yoga class would give them the chance to chat.

Polly was sitting on the hotel balcony at a table covered with a crisp linen tablecloth, enjoying a breakfast of fresh pineapple and papaya while gazing out over a sparkling, turquoise bay. Simon had just taken a shower and walked out onto the balcony wrapped up in a white towelling robe. He looked wonderful, and Polly had never felt happier. London, her City job and Harry all seemed a world away. 'I've organized a day out on a speed boat for us, we're leaving at 10.30 so there's no need to rush,' he said as he stroked her hair. 'Then tonight we're having dinner at a rather special seafood restaurant one of the other guests recommended to me. It's in the next bay along from the hotel, looking out over a deserted beach.'

Back in their minimalist hotel room after a sun-drenched day on the boat, Polly washed the salt and suntan lotion out of her hair and thought about what she was going to wear for dinner. She wanted to look chic but relaxed, so she pulled a turquoise dress out of the wardrobe and slipped on some kitten-heel mules. Her golden skin looked fantastic against the turquoise of her dress. She spritzed a little volumizing spray through her hair, relieved that she had remembered to buy some mini-sized hair products in the airport before the flight. Polly then blow-dried her hair with a curling brush to put some volume into her blonde locks, before twisting her hair up into a casual but so chic chignon. She pinned her hair into place and looked at herself in the mirror. A dash of bronzing powder across her cheeks, a little sparkly eye-shadow, mascara and soft pink lip gloss were all she needed to enhance her healthy glow. She was ready for her evening with Simon.

After a short drive along the coastline, Polly and Simon were seated at a secluded table looking out over the golden sand. Simon ordered a bottle of Champagne, raised his glass to toast their evening and then reached across the table for Polly's hand. 'Polly,' he said, looking serious, 'I've got something I want to talk to you about …'

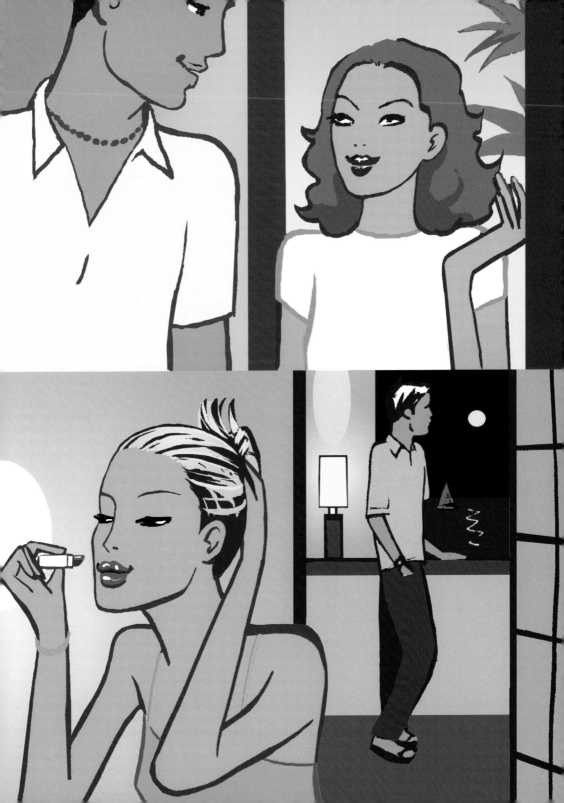

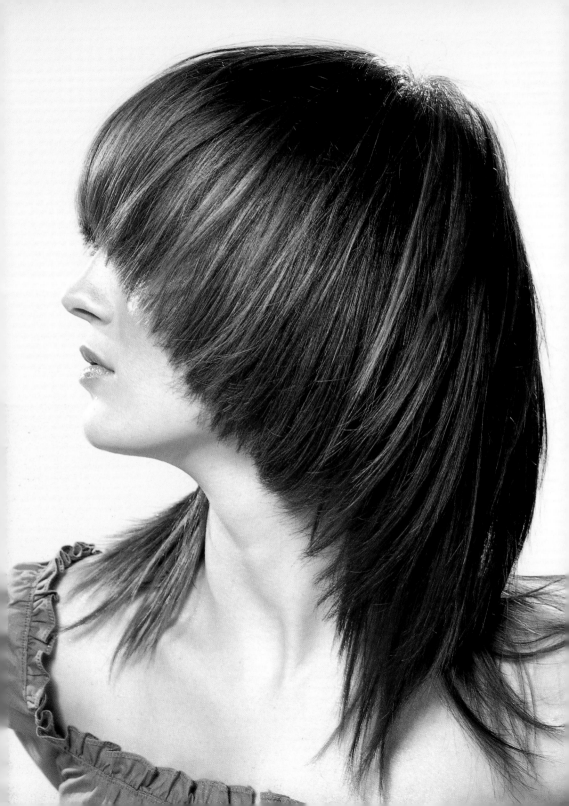

SOS hair repair

If you are concerned in any way about your hair once you get back from your holiday, go to your hair salon for a consultation. This is normally free of charge and gives you the chance to talk through the condition, cut and colour of your hair with your stylist and colourist so that they can advise the best plan of action for post-holiday haircare.

cut

The quickest way to get holiday hair back into condition is to cut out all the dry, split ends that leave it looking dull. Once hair has been cut back into shape, it will look sleek and shiny without much extra effort. Remember to book an appointment before you go away, so that you can dash into the salon on your return. If your hair is dry and damaged, your stylist may have to cut away up to 1 cm (½ inch) to get it back into condition. But if you've spent time conditioning your hair while you were away and it's in good shape on your return, your stylist can just snip away the split ends without taking any length off your hair.

colour

Once you are back from holiday, continue to treat your hair with conditioning treatments. This will even out porosity, maintain the condition and ensure that your next colour treatment takes evenly. Give your hair a weekly detox shampoo to remove the build-up of chlorine and salt water on the hair shaft. Have a good look at your colour once you get home. You may love the sun-kissed highlights around your face and on the tips of your hair, so take a photograph of it. That way, your colourist has a reference and can re-create the look if you want holiday glamour put back into your hair at a later date. If your hair has gone too light, your colourist can add some deeper lowlights or apply a colour gloss to tone down the overall colour, make it look more natural or take it back to the colour it was before your trip.

holiday tips for coloured hair

A great way to start a hair-repair regime is with a scalp and head massage, as it stimulates the secretion of natural, moisturizing oils.

Use a cleansing detox shampoo, which leaves the hair ultra-clean and revitalized, then apply a deep-conditioning treatment to replace moisture and even out the porosity of the hair.

Colour glossing treatments rejuvenate hair colour, and add shine and condition, without drying it out.

There are products that help prevent colour fade, so splash out on these before you go away – it'll be cheaper than a repair job when you return.

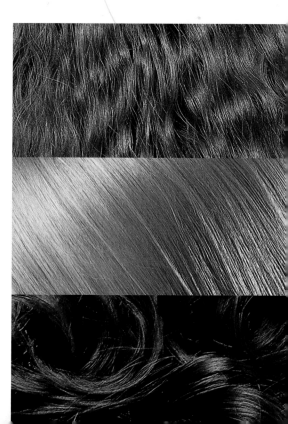

Back from their holiday, Jaz and Chrissie are feeling far from refreshed and rejuvenated. They have partied through the night and sunned themselves on the beach all day long for the entire week, and are now well and truly in need of a post-holiday overhaul. They're sitting in the kitchen assessing the damage. Chrissie has overdone the sunbathing and she's suffering the consequences – she's burnt her scalp, her hair looks dry and brittle, and she's beginning to peel around her hairline. Jaz is worried about split ends. Despite her careful attempts to protect her hair, all the heat from the sun, together with her nightly hairstyling regime has left the ends dry. 'Let's finish off our holiday with a pampering session,' says Jaz. 'We've spent so much already, a little extra on a trip to the salon won't hurt,' agrees Chrissie. 'Great tans, girls,' says Charles as he greets them at the salon. 'But your hair is in distress!' 'Do whatever you can,' sighs Jaz, as the girls sit down in front of the mirrors for their consultations. Charles decides that both girls need to have an intensive deep-conditioning treatment to put the moisture

... jaz's and chrissie's bad-hair day

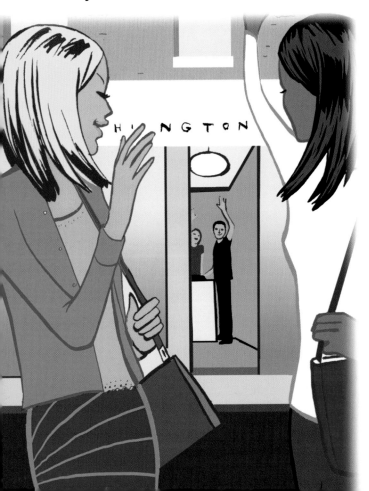

back into their hair and revitalize the condition. Then he cuts just the ends off Jaz's hair to get rid of all the split ends without losing the length. Chrissie finds that she needs to have a bit more taken off her hair as the ends have got so dry. 'You need to have some honey-blonde tints put through your hair Chrissie,' says her colourist, Carolyn. 'Your hair's been bleached by the sun and it's too hard on your skin tone,' she advises. 'I'm in your hands,' says Chrissie.

Three hours later, Jaz and Chrissie leave the salon feeling more rested than they have in the whole of the last week. Their hair is looking sleek, glossy and full of body. 'We should do this more often,' says Chrissie as they head for a designer clothes shop for a spot of window shopping. 'I think I could just about get used to it,' laughs Jaz.

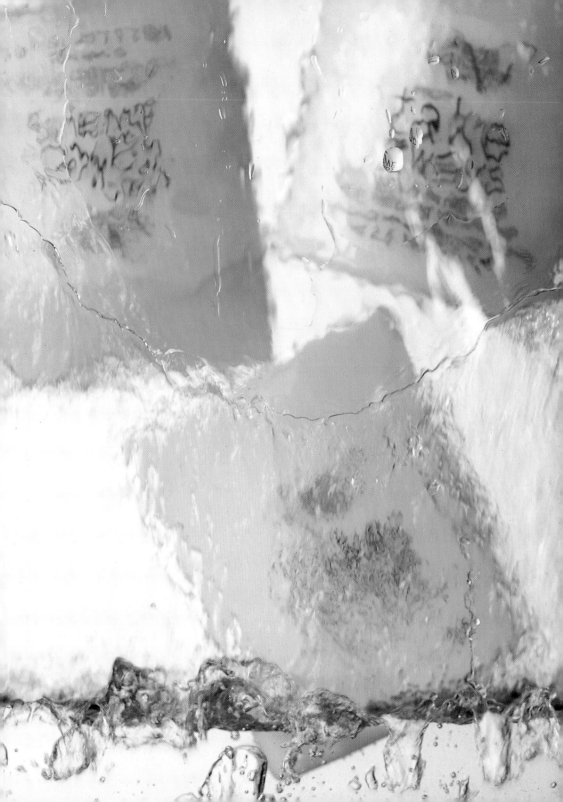

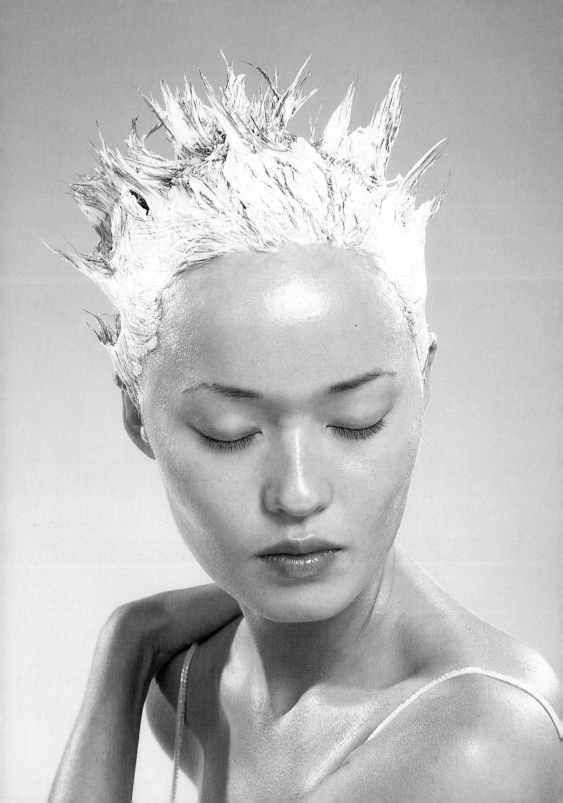

hair treats

There are a number of really effective treatments you can use to replenish the moisture levels of dehydrated hair, encourage growth, improve strength and flexibility and restore shine and gloss. You can book in for a treatment at your salon on your return, do it at home, or, even better, while you are on holiday to help maintain condition and prevent damage from occurring.

scalp treatment

As its name suggests, this treatment stimulates and revitalizes the skin of the scalp for better, stronger hair growth. It is usually made up of soothing and moisturizing ingredients that help to prevent itching, flaking and general discomfort. It will encourage the growth of new hair by nourishing the roots and it also conditions the hair shaft. Scalp treatments are good for all hair types, particularly if the scalp is burnt or dry after a holiday.

conditioning mask

Designed to be left on the hair for between 3 and 20 minutes, a conditioning mask will hydrate the hair shaft with moisturizing ingredients and nourish the hair and scalp without causing heaviness. Conditioning masks are designed to work most effectively on the damaged or dehydrated areas of the hair, leaving it nourished and protected. This is a good treatment to use during your holiday and on your return, whatever your hair type.

deep-conditioning treatment

More intensive than a conditioning mask, this hair treatment literally gets to the root of the problem by nourishing the scalp as well as the hair itself. It homes in on damaged areas and delivers intensive moisture exactly where it's needed. This extra-rich treatment is best for extremely dry and parched hair.

hair detox

A deep-cleansing shampoo that removes the build-up of dirt, styling products and pollutants from the hair, without stripping it or leaving it dry. This is especially useful if your hair is looking dull after a holiday or for colour-treated hair that might need a revitalizing boost.

nutrition

Diet plays a huge part in the health of our hair, and a holiday is a great time to eat well and boost the body's vitality with good nutrition. The sure-fire way to make your hair limp and thin is to skip meals or eat badly. So what do you need to eat?

diet tips

Do not crash diet before you go away, as this puts strain on the system and deprives your body of essential nutrients – the first to suffer will be your hair.

A balanced wholefood diet, with essential fats, plenty of carbohydrates, protein and fresh fruit and vegetables will keep your hair healthy and shiny.

The best sources of essential fats are oily fish, such as sardines and salmon, and vegetable oils, such as olive and linseed (flax); these will help to keep the skin and hair in good condition.

Eat plenty of carbohydrates such as brown rice, wholewheat pasta, pulses and lentils.

Fresh fruit, vegetables and salads provide antioxidant vitamins, which help prevent premature ageing in the body and the hair.

Since the hair is made up of protein, you need to keep your protein levels high by means of your diet. Fish, chicken, meat and eggs all provide the best proteins, although other sources such as nuts, cereals, milk and cheese will also supplement your intake.

hair supplements

A good daily multivitamin will give you the balance of vitamins and minerals that your body and hair need to keep them in optimum condition. The condition of your hair will be boosted by all the B vitamins, gamma-linolenic acid (GLA), fish oil, linseed (flax) oil, antioxidant vitamins including beta-carotene, vitamins C and E, and the minerals selenium and zinc.

Back at home again, Kate decides to spend spend the last few hours of her holiday relaxing. She has a long shower and then applies a conditioning hair mask to her hair, twists a small towel into a turban on her head and wraps herself up in her dressing gown. Kate makes a cup of tea and then, feeling wonderfully relaxed, she settles down on the sofa to watch a video.

Next morning, Kate wakes early and performs her new ritual of yoga stretches before breakfast. Getting ready for work, she takes a good look at herself in the mirror. Her lightly tanned, glowing skin needs little make-up, so she sticks to mascara and a touch of bronzer. Her curly hair is looking glossy and healthy with flattering golden streaks from the sun. She decides to leave it natural and

simply works some styling cream through the ends to give the curls extra definition. Work, and most importantly Matthew, will have to take her as they find her. If two weeks at the yoga retreat have taught her anything, it's to have the confidence to be herself. Her Miss-Get-Ahead-At-Work act has got her nowhere – perhaps her new-found contentment and inner strength will do the trick.

... kate returns home from India

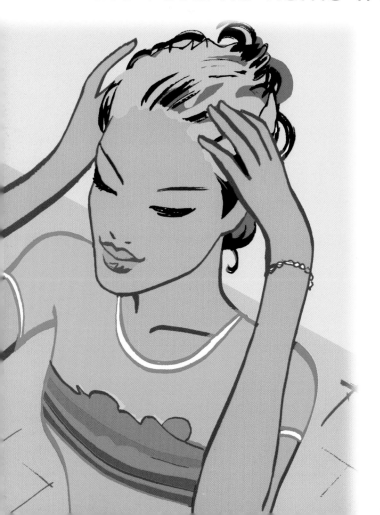

An hour later she walks into the office, makes herself a cup of green tea and sits down at her desk to check her e-mails. Matthew walks past her desk and then stops suddenly.
'Kate, I hardly recognized you,' he gasps. His expression changes from surprise to pleasure.
'You're looking fabulous – where did you go again?' he asks.
'You'd know if you'd bothered to ask,' thinks Kate to herself.
'India,' she replies brightly.
'Well, it's obviously agreed with you,' Matthew says, looking her up and down. Keeping his eyes fixed on Kate as he hands her some paperwork, he suggests they go out for lunch so he can fill her in on the latest marketing project.
'Sure,' Kate replies calmly.
She turns back to her computer, and there in her e-mail inbox is a message from Luke. 'Got the job at The Yoga Centre in Notting Hill. Will be back in two months. Missing you,' it said.

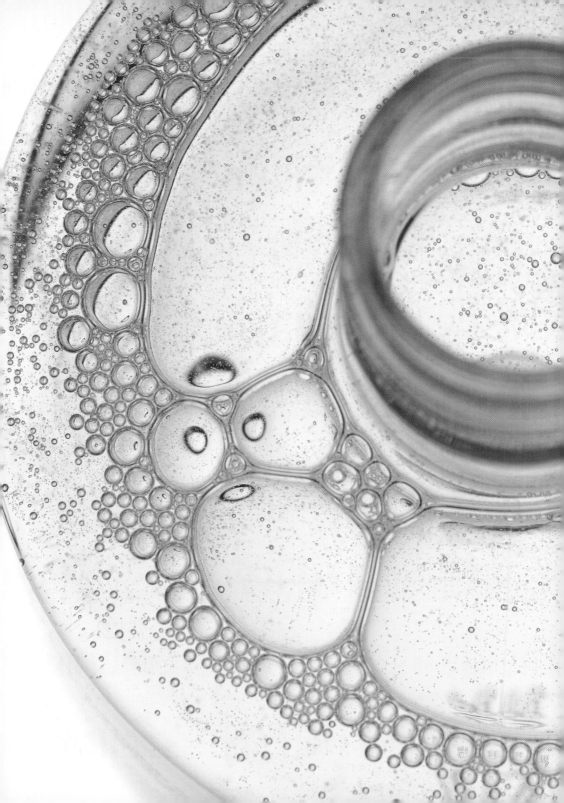

hair doctor

my blonde hair looks distinctly green after my holiday. Is there anything I can do?

The reason your hair can go green is because of the blue dye that is used to show up the chlorine in swimming pools (chlorine is, in fact, clear). Highlights make your hair more porous than usual and so the blue dye can penetrate the hair shaft and react with the highlighting chemicals in your hair. Try using a detox shampoo designed to thoroughly but gently cleanse the hair. Or, try applying concentrated tomato juice or tomato ketchup to the hair, as the red colouring should neutralize any green in your hair. If the green tinge to your hair will not budge, you need to go to a hair salon where the stylist will 'deep cleanse' your hair with a mild pre-lightening agent to lift out the colour. Your colourist will then freshen up your original colour.

my hair seems dull, lacklustre and flat after my week away. Why is it looking so bad?

It is possible that your hair has been beaten by the combination of sun damage, chlorine or salt and, if you have been using styling products that contain silica, a build-up of product on your hair. On your return from holiday, use a clarifying shampoo to remove deep deposits of dirt and the build-up of styling products. Then book yourself into your salon and ask your stylist to trim off all the split ends – the result is immediate. Your hair will look sharp, clean and sleek. Your stylist may also recommend that you have a revitalizing hair treatment while you are in the salon, but the combination of simple cut and condition should do the trick.

my scalp is dry and flaky after my holiday. Do I have dandruff?

It's more than likely that you have burnt your scalp in the sun while you were away and the skin on your scalp is peeling. Dandruff tends to be more common among people who have oily hair, not a dry scalp. So if you have post-holiday flakes, visit your hair salon for an intensive deep-conditioning treatment that includes a scalp treatment to feed the hair as well as soothe and rehydrate the skin on your head. Don't rush for the nearest anti-dandruff shampoo unless the problem persists well after your return. If, after a few weeks, you still see flakes in your hairline, try using an anti-dandruff shampoo every other day. When lathered up, remember to leave the shampoo on for a few minutes to allow the ingredients to work, moisturizing and exfoliating the scalp. Alternate anti-dandruff shampoo with your usual shampoo until the problem clears.

if I wash my hair every day on holiday, will it be more oily when I return home?

It is one of the big haircare myths that washing your hair every day will make it oilier. Using a gentle, daily shampoo will not leave your hair more oily or stimulate the sebum glands on your scalp to produce more oil. More importantly, washing out the cocktail of haircare products, salt and chlorine that usually comes with a break away and putting the moisture back into your hair at the end of each day with a good conditioner will leave your hair glossy, well conditioned and healthy.

the ends of my hair seem really dry. Can I use a product to repair my split ends?

Any product that is designed to treat split ends offers only a temporary, cosmetic solution. Split-end products and hairsprays simply hold the ends together until either the hair is brushed vigorously or washed. The only way to get rid of post-holiday split ends is to have them cut off. Your hairstylist will be able to snip the ends away without taking a great length off your hair, provided that you have kept your hair in good condition while you were away.

if I use lemon on my hair while I sunbathe is it a 'natural' way to give me highlights?

Lemon juice may help to bleach hair in the sun as the juice is acidic (although how effective it is remains debatable). But be warned: neat lemon juice is extremely damaging to the hair. It will dry it out while you lie in the sun and your scalp may be left sore and sun-sensitive. The sun will fade your hair colour in a hot climate and this bleaching action damages your hair as it weakens the structure of the cells and causes permanent damage. It's best to forget about lemon juice and leave it to your hair colourist to change your colour and add highlights.

polly's big announcement

The girls were all back from their globe-trotting and, at Polly's request, were having a night in together. Her sitting room was filled with excited chatter as they caught up on each other's news. Polly had called from the office to say that she would have to work until 8.30 but that she would bring supper with her. She had to put in some extra time after her break in the Seychelles with Simon in case anyone at her City firm thought she wasn't taking her job seriously.

'I'm going to open a bottle of wine – does anyone want a glass while we wait for Polly?' asked Jaz.

'Yes, and grab some crisps while you're at it,' ordered Chrissie, who was curled up on the floor painting her toenails with iridescent pink varnish. 'So you survived the jungle and John?' she said sarcastically to Laura, who was showing Kate her photographs of river rafting and orang-utan in the jungle's nature reserve.

'It was incredible,' replied Laura, who was very happily reliving the trip. 'John's thinking of moving into nature documentaries. We were both so taken with the wildlife and we want to raise awareness for the conservation work that needs to be done in the jungle,' she said.

'So you'd actually consider living out there for months, with all those huge insects?' asked Chrissie, shuddering visibly.

'Well, I can see how you'd have a problem living without your kitten heels and your hairdryer,' laughed Kate, 'but Laura's pretty resourceful.'

'I'm home,' yelled Polly, as she headed for the kitchen with a bag full of Thai takeaway. 'Come and have some food while it's hot,' she called to the girls.

'I've got green curry, rice and steamed vegetables,' she said as they gathered round. They each grabbed a bowl of food and took it back into the sitting room. 'Champagne?' asked Polly as she joined them with a large, chilled bottle and glasses.

'This is pushing the boat out a bit isn't it?' said Laura.

'Well, it seems to me that we've got things to celebrate,' said Polly, handing the girls a glass each. Polly raised her glass in the air. 'Here's to Jaz's new job in the fashion world, and to Laura and John's new venture – let's hope it works out.' The girls toasted their future as they drank.

'So let's hear about the Seychelles and Simon,' demanded Chrissie. An uncontrollable smile spread instantly across Polly's face.

'You really like him, don't you Polly?' asked Kate.

'He's just perfect. We had the most incredible time and the thing is, well, he's asked me to marry him,' Polly burst out excitedly. There was a moment's stunned silence before the girls shrieked in unison.

'Marry him?' gasped Laura. 'Polly, that's so quick.'

'I know it seems like a whirlwind romance,' agreed Polly. 'I've only known him for a few months but we both know it's right and we can't see the point in hanging around and waiting. I was hoping you would all be there for me – as my bridesmaids.'

'Of course we will,' answered Laura quickly.

'Now tell us about the ring – have you chosen a huge stone?' asked Chrissie, true to form.

The rest of the evening was filled with wedding talk as the girls debated what Polly should wear, laughed about hideous meringue dresses and discussed how they should have their hair. Life at 23 Havana Road had certainly moved on fast.

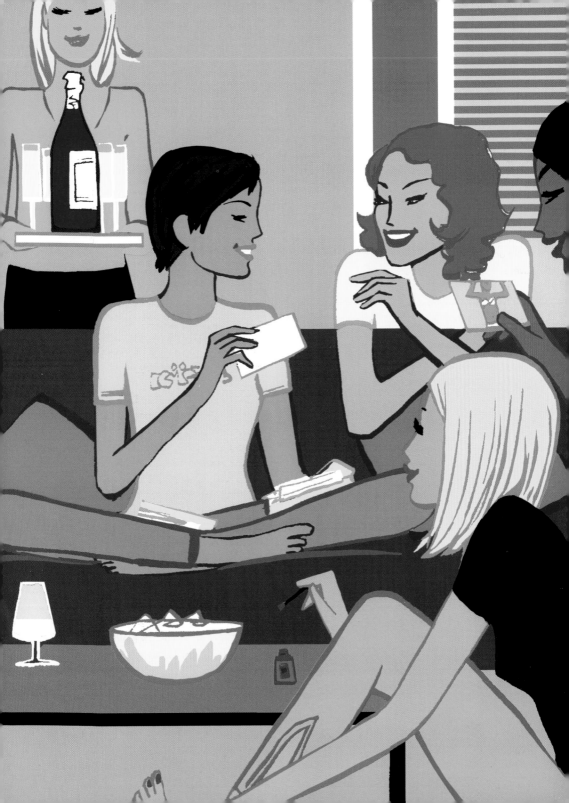

acknowledgements

Thank you to Adam Reed and Carolyn Newman
at the Percy Street salon. With special thanks to
Julie Gibson Jarvie, Penny Stock and Venetia Penfold,
without whom the book wouldn't have been possible.

With special thanks to the following:

Bud (by appointment only), tel: 020 8537 0626

Butler & Wilson, 20 South Molten Street, London W1K 5QY,
tel: 020 7409 2955